Get ahead!
medicine
300 SBAs for finals

Get ahead!

medicine
300 SBAs for finals

Series Editor:
Saran Shantikumar MD Academic Clinical
Fellow in Surgery, Nuffield Department of
Surgery, John Radcliffe Hospital, Oxford, UK

Authors:
Benjamin McNeillis BA BM BCʜ F2 Doctor, Oxford
Deanery, John Radcliffe Hospital, Oxford, UK

Rhian James MA (Hons) BM BCʜɪʀ F2 Doctor,
Heatherwood and Wexham Park Hospital Trust,
Slough, UK

Ai Ling Koh MB CʜB F2 Doctor, Oxford Deanery,
Wexham Park Hospital, Slough, UK

Tim Sparkes MBBS BEɴɢ F2 Doctor, Oxford
Deanery, John Radcliffe Hospital, Oxford, UK

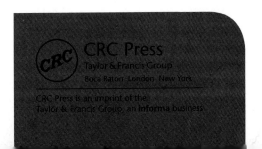

CRC Press
Taylor & Francis Group
Boca Raton London New York

CRC Press is an imprint of the
Taylor & Francis Group, an informa business

CRC Press
Taylor & Francis Group
6000 Broken Sound Parkway NW, Suite 300
Boca Raton, FL 33487-2742

© 2012 by Taylor & Francis Group, LLC
CRC Press is an imprint of Taylor & Francis Group, an Informa business

Printed and bound in Great Britain by CPI Group (UK) Ltd, Croydon, CR0 4YY

No claim to original U.S. Government works

Visit the Taylor & Francis Web site at
http://www.taylorandfrancis.com

and the CRC Press Web site at
http://www.crcpress.com

Contents

Preface

Welcome to *Get ahead! Medicine*. This book contains 300 Single Best Answer (SBA) questions covering various topics within clinical surgery. The SBAs are arranged as six practice papers, each containing 50 questions. Allow yourself 60–90 minutes for each paper. You can either work through the practice papers systematically or dip in and out of the book using the SBA index as a guide to where questions on a specific topic can be found. We have tried to include all the main conditions about which you can be expected to know, as well as some more detailed knowledge suitable for candidates aiming towards distinction. As in the real exam, these papers have no preset pass mark. Whether you pass or fail depends on the distribution of scores across the whole year group, but around 60% should be sufficient.

We hope this book fulfils its aim in being a useful, informative revision aid. If you have any feedback or suggestions, please let us know (RevisionForMedicalFinals@gmail.com).

We would like to acknowledge the help of Sarah Vasey, Jo Koster and Sarah Penny of Hodder Arnold, for their guidance, support and patience throughout this project.

Ben McNeillis
Rhian James
Ai Ling Koh
Tim Sparkes
Saran Shantikumar

Introduction to Get Ahead Medicine

GET AHEAD!

Single Best Answer questions (SBAs) are becoming more popular as a method of assessment in summative medical school examinations. Each clinical vignette is followed by a list of five possible answers, of which only one is correct. SBAs have the advantage of testing candidates' knowledge of clinical scenarios rather than their ability at detailed factual recall. They do not always parallel real-life situations, however, and are no comparison to clinical decision making. Either way the SBA is here to stay.

The *Get ahead!* series is aimed primarily at undergraduate finalists. Much like the real exam we have endeavoured to include commonly asked questions as well as a generous proportion of harder stems, appropriate for the more ambitious student aiming for honours. The Universities Medical Assessment Partnership (UMAP) is a collaboration of 14 medical schools in the UK, which is compiling a bank of SBAs and EMQs to be used in summative examinations. The questions in the *Get ahead!* series are written to closely follow the 'house style' of the UMAP SBAs, and hence are of a similar format to what many of you can expect in your exams. All the questions in the *Get ahead!* series are accompanied by explanatory answers including a succinct summary of the key features of each condition. Even when you get an answer right I strongly suggest you read these – I guarantee you'll learn something. For added interest we have included details of eponymous persons ('eponymous' from Greek *epi* = upon + *onyma* = name; 'giving name') and, as you have just seen, some derivations of words from the original Latin or Greek.

HOW TO PASS YOUR EXAMS

The clinical scenarios given in SBAs are intended to be based on 'house officer knowledge'. Sadly this is not always the case and you shouldn't be surprised when you get a question concerning the underlying histology of testicular tumours (as I was). So start revising early and don't restrict yourself to the given syllabus if you can avoid it. If your exam is only 2 weeks away then CRAM, CRAM, CRAM – you'll be surprised at how much you can learn in a fortnight.

DURING THE EXAM

1. Try to answer the questions without looking at the responses at first – the questions are written such that this should be possible.
2. Take your time to read the questions fully. There are no bonus marks available for finishing the paper early.

3. If you get stuck on a question then make sure you mark down your best guess before you move on. You may not have time to come back to it at the end.

4. Answer all the questions – there is no negative marking. If you are unsure go with your instinct – it's probably going to be your best guess.

5. Never think that the examiner is trying to catch you out. Red herrings are not allowed so don't assume there is one. If a question looks easy it probably is!

This is obvious: there is no substitute for learning the material thoroughly and practising as many questions as you can. With this book you're off to a good start!

A FINAL WORD

The *Get ahead!* series is written by junior doctors who have recently finished finals and who have experience teaching students. As such, I hope the books cover information that is valuable and relevant to you as undergraduates who are about to sit finals.

I wish you the best of luck in your exams!

Saran Shantikumar
Series editor, *Get ahead!*

Practice Paper 1: Questions

1. Acute coronary syndrome (1)

In the treatment of acute coronary syndrome (ACS), which of the following statements is FALSE?

A Aspirin and clopidogrel do not provide enough anticoagulation; heparin should also be given

B Give 75 mg aspirin *stat*

C Give 300 mg clopidogrel in addition to aspirin

D Hypotension, asthma and bradycardia are the main contraindicators to beta blockade

E Patients will likely continue taking a statin, beta-blocker and angiotensin-converting enzyme (ACE) inhibitor on discharge home

2. Obstructive renal impairment

Which of the following is not a potential cause of obstructive renal impairment?

A Benign prostatic hypertrophy

B Recurrent kidney stones

C Retroperitoneal fibrosis

D Schistosomiasis

E Systemic sclerosis

3. Management of skin lesions (1)

A 60-year-old man who works for an oil company presents with a lesion on the temple that is bothering him as it is growing. It bled once when he knocked it. On examination, the lesion is 8 mm in diameter and is a flat, mildly erythematous patch with a few scales and a larger keratotic horn in the centre. There are no other lesions on inspection of his skin and no personal or family history of skin cancer.

Which of the following is the most appropriate management plan?

A Cryotherapy

B Curettage

C Excisional biopsy

D Topical 5-fluorouracil

E Wide local excision

4. Chest X-ray

A 68-year-old man who is recently diagnosed with lung cancer is admitted to the emergency department with acute shortness of breath. A chest X-ray shows a right upper zone (RUZ) collapse.

What do you expect to find on examination?

	Trachea	Percussion	Auscultation
A	Deviated to right	Dull RUZ	Reduced breath sounds
B	Deviated to right	Dull RUZ	Wheeze
C	Deviated to right	Resonant RUZ	Reduced breath sounds
D	Deviated to left	Dull RUZ	Reduced breath sounds
E	Deviated to left	Resonant RUZ	Wheeze

5. Headaches

A 68-year-old woman presents to her GP with headaches and visual disturbance. She has also noticed that she gets an itchy rash when she gets out of a hot bath. On examination she has a ruddy complexion and a palpable spleen. Her only previous medical history is gout. Initial blood tests reveal a raised packed red cell volume with a raised red cell mass, along with a raised white cell count and thrombocytosis.

What is the most likely diagnosis?

A Chronic myeloid leukaemia
B Lymphoma
C Migraine with aura
D Polycythaemia rubra vera
E Soap allergy

6. Chronic obstructive pulmonary disease

A 45-year-old man who is a heavy smoker is recently diagnosed with chronic obstructive pulmonary disease (COPD). He has no documented acute exacerbations in the past.

Which of the following treatment is NOT suitable in the management of COPD in this patient?

A Annual influenza and pneumococcal vaccination
B Inhaled corticosteroids
C Short-acting β2-agonist
D Short-acting anti-cholinergic
E Smoking cessation

7. Management of asthma (1)

A 35-year-old woman is admitted to hospital with quick-onset shortness of breath. She has a past medical history of asthma. Her observations include a pulse rate 120 bpm, blood pressure 100/72 mmHg, respiratory rate 30/

min and SaO$_2$ 88% on room air. On examination, she appears to be drowsy and exhausted. Her chest is quiet on auscultation. Arterial blood gases show: pH 7.35, PaO$_2$ 5.2 kPa, PaCO$_2$ 4.9 kPa and bicarbonate 24 mmol/L.

Which of the following would NOT be appropriate in the management of this case?

A High-flow oxygen
B High-dose nebulised beta-2 agonists
C Intravenous magnesium sulphate
D Leukotriene receptor antagonists
E Steroids

8. Collapse (1)

A 19-year-old footballer has collapsed on the pitch. His airway is clear and he is brought to the emergency department, where he begins to recover and denies that he has chest pain. He has never had anything like this before.

Which of the following is the most likely diagnosis?

A Carotid stenosis
B Hypertrophic obstructive cardiomyopathy (HOCM)
C Myocardial infarction
D Rheumatic fever
E Thyrotoxicosis

9. Eczema versus psoriasis

A 31-year-old man presents to your clinic with a year-long history of itchy red scaly lesions.

Which of the following would make you more likely to diagnose eczema rather than psoriasis?

A Associated nail changes
B History of distal interphalangeal joint pain and swelling
C Localised to flexures rather than extensors
D Well-demarcated lesions
E Worsening in winter months

10. Diagnosis of multiple sclerosis (1)

Which of the following best describes the MRI findings in multiple sclerosis?

A Cortical grey matter inflammatory lesions
B Longitudinally extensive transverse myelitis (more than three spinal segments)
C Periventricular white matter lesions matching the clinical picture
D Periventricular white matter lesions not necessarily matching the clinical picture
E White matter lesions exclusively in the cerebellum and brainstem

11. The multidisciplinary team

A 67-year-old man is discharged from hospital following an incision and drainage of a large abdominal wall abscess. He needs someone to help change his wound packing regularly, however he is immobile and lives alone.

Which member of the multidisciplinary team would be most appropriate to help?

A District nurse
B Health visitor
C Occupational therapist
D Orthotist
E Social worker

12. Diagnosis of chest pain (1)

A 69-year-old man presents to the emergency department with ongoing chest pain. He has a past medical history of intermittent claudication and hypertension. He is an overweight smoker and heavy drinker of alcohol. On analysing the electrocardiogram (ECG), you notice broad S-waves in the right-hand chest leads, two R-waves per complex in the left-hand chest leads and ST-segment elevation. He asks if he has had a heart attack.

What is the best answer to this question?

A No – but we need to do more tests to find the true cause
B No – it's just right bundle branch block
C No – it's just angina
D Yes
E I'm not sure; we need to do more tests

13. Risk factors for ischaemic heart disease

Which of the following is not a preventable risk factor for coronary artery disease?

A Five cigarettes per day smoking history
B High low-density lipoprotein (LDL) cholesterol levels
C Hypertension
D Obesity
E 12 U/week alcohol history

14. Diagnosis of cough (1)

A 29-year-old man presents to the emergency department with a 1-week history of non-productive cough, muscle aches, fever, vomiting and diarrhoea. His observations include temperature 38.4°C, pulse rate 105 bpm, blood pressure 110/76 mmHg and respiratory rate 22/min. On examination, his chest is clear to both auscultation and percussion. A chest X-ray shows bilateral lung basal infiltrates. The blood results show Na+ 128 mmol/L, K+ 4.0 mmol/L, urea 5.9 mmol/L, creatinine 130 μmol/L, albumin 26 g/L, ALT 106 IU/L, ALP 230 IU/L.

What is the most likely causative organism?

A *Chlamydia pneumoniae*
B *Mycoplasma pneumoniae*
C *Legionella pneumophila*
D *Staphylococcus aureus*
E *Streptococcus pneumoniae*

15. Diagnosis of vertigo

A 60-year-old man presents with a history of recurrent dizzy spells for the past 4 months, which occur daily. The dizzy spells last a few minutes and seem to occur if he moves his head, as a result of which he keeps his head as still as possible. The attacks are not associated with any deafness or tinnitus and a neurological examination is entirely normal. You favour a diagnosis of benign paroxysmal positional vertigo.

Which of the following descriptions of findings on Hallpike's manoeuvre would confirm this diagnosis?

A Delayed onset (a few seconds) torsional nystagmus on descent facing both sides
B Delayed onset (a few seconds) torsional nystagmus on descent facing one side only
C Immediate torsional nystagmus on descent facing both sides
D Immediate torsional nystagmus on descent facing one side only
E No nystagmus on descent facing either side

16. Epistaxis

A 43-year-old man presents to his GP with a 3-month history of recurrent nose bleeds, mucosal bleeding, haemoptysis and recurrent sinusitis. Besides that, he also noticed that he has increasingly become short of breath. On examination, he had a nasal deformity and chest auscultation revealed crackles in the left lower zone. A urine dipstick test showed microscopic haematuria.

Which of the following is the most likely diagnosis?

A Chronic myeloid leukaemia
B Chronic lymphocytic leukaemia
C Churg–Strauss syndrome
D Goodpasture syndrome
E Wegener granulomatosis

17. Diarrhoea (1)

Following a protracted stay in hospital following a severe chest infection, an 83-year-old man develops bloody diarrhoea.

What is the most likely cause?

A Adenocarcinoma of the bowel
B *Clostridium difficile* infection
C Norovirus infection
D *Salmonella* infection
E *Shigella* infection

18. Diagnosis of malaria

A 21-year-old student on an internship with *The Guardian* travel section has recently returned from a backpacking holiday in West Africa. For the last few days he has been having headaches, flu-like symptoms and muscle aches, and now he has started rigoring.

Which investigation should be performed to rule out malaria?

A Blood cultures
B Falciparum antigen dipstick test
C Liver biopsy
D One blood film
E Three thick and thin blood films on consecutive days

19. Electrocardiogram (1)

You are asked to review an electrocardiogram (ECG) in the emergency department. Helpfully, a summary of details is printed at the top as follows: rate 88/min, regular rhythm, axis −20°, PR duration 0.26 seconds (constant), QRS complex 0.08 seconds, QT interval 0.2 seconds. You note that P-waves are only present before each QRS and that the rhythm is regular.

Which of the following would be the best summary?

A First-degree heart block
B Left axis deviation
C Left bundle branch block
D Refuse to summarise until it can be compared with an old ECG
E Ventricular tachycardia

20. Investigation of deranged liver function tests

A 65-year-old man with a longstanding diagnosis of chronic obstructive pulmonary disease has been reviewed by his GP for deteriorating liver function tests and clinical signs and symptoms of cirrhosis.

What investigation should the GP arrange?

A Alpha-1-antitrypsin serum levels
B Alpha-feto protein levels
C Anti-smooth muscle antibodies
D Gamma GT levels
E Hepatitis screen

21. Epigastric pain (1)

A 44-year-old woman presents to the emergency department with pain. The pain is epigastric, sharp in nature, worse on lying flat and during inspiration. She has recently suffered a chest infection. She is not a smoker. On examination, she has diffuse inspiratory crepitations. Her oxygen saturation is 98% on room air. Her ECG shows widespread saddle-shaped ST elevation.

Which of the following is the most likely diagnosis?

A Acute pericarditis
B Angina
C Myocardial infarction
D Pleurisy
E Pulmonary embolism

22. Gout prophylaxis

A 55-year-old overweight pub landlord presents with a several-year history of episodic acute painful joint swelling that started in his left big toe and now affects his knees. Symptoms improve with use of diclofenac. Gout was diagnosed on his first hospital visit, however this now appears recurrent. He developed an acute attack in his left knee 2 days ago.

Which of the following represents the best plan for prophylaxis?

A Keep on long-term diclofenac with gastric protection
B Start allopurinol now with non-steroidal anti-inflammatory drugs (NSAIDs) cover and increase until his urate is below 300 μmol/L
C Start allopurinol at least 2 weeks after the acute attack has settled with NSAID cover and increase until his urate level is below 300 μmol/L
D Switch to long-term colchicine
E Switch to use of depot steroid injections

23. Hepatomegaly

Which of the following conditions does not classically cause hepatomegaly?

A End-stage cirrhosis
B Fatty liver
C Hepatocellular carcinoma
D Myeloproliferative disease
E Right-sided heart failure

24. Sclerosing cholangitis

Which of the following conditions is associated with sclerosing cholangitis?

A Autoimmune hepatitis
B Coeliac disease
C Irritable bowel syndrome
D Pernicious anaemia
E Ulcerative colitis (UC)

25. Investigation of status epilepticus

A 35-year-old homeless man presents to the emergency department in a state of unconsciousness. He was fitting when the ambulance crew got to him 20 minutes ago, and a friend at the scene estimated that he had started fitting "around 15 minutes before". His friend informed the ambulance crew that he is a known epileptic and you find a pack of phenytoin on him. He looks dishevelled and smells of alcohol. He has a blood pressure of 170/95 mmHg and temperature 37.9°C. On examination there is a quiet systolic murmur, though it is difficult to fully characterise.

Which of the following investigations will be most useful at this stage?

A Computed tomography (CT) of the brain
B Echocardiogram
C Electroencephalogram (EEG)
D Magnetic resonance imaging (MRI) of the brain
E Phenytoin levels

26. Shortness of breath (1)

A 74-year-old male ex-comedian can no longer perform at smoky open-microphone nights due to shortness of breath. He is coughing up frothy white sputum, which recently has contained a small amount of blood. On examination, his chest demonstrates diffuse crackles on inspiration through which you can just discern a mid-diastolic murmur and a loud first heart sound. His chest X-ray confirms pulmonary oedema.

What is the most likely underlying cause for his symptoms?

A Lower respiratory tract infection
B Mitral stenosis
C Non-small cell carcinoma of the lung
D Pulmonary embolism
E Small cell carcinoma of the lung

27. Aortic regurgitation

In clinic, a retired 62-year-old man presents with shortness of breath on exertion. You find a collapsing pulse and subsequent echocardiography confirms aortic regurgitation.

Which of the following is NOT associated with aortic regurgitation?

A Ankylosing spondylosis
B Aortic dissection
C Marfan syndrome
D Rheumatic fever
E Systemic lupus erythematosus (SLE)

28. Management of oliguria (1)

A previously fit and well 70-year-old woman has been admitted due to a fractured neck of femur, and she has recently returned to the ward after a cemented hemiarthroplasty. You are bleeped to the ward to see her, as it is noted that she has had only 30 ml urine output in the last 3 hours. She is asleep on the ward, with a patient-controlled analgesic device *in situ*. Her airway is intact and her respiratory rate is 12/min with normal saturations and good air entry bilaterally. Her pulse is 125 bpm with a blood pressure of 95/68 mmHg and she has delayed capillary refill. She has pale conjunctiva and a temperature of 37.3°C. She has a 12-hourly bag of normal saline running. Her catheter is draining concentrated urine. An abdominal examination is normal.

Which of the following interventions would you try first to increase the urine output?

A Fluid challenge of 500 ml 5% dextrose over 10 minutes
B Fluid challenge of 500 ml normal saline over 10 minutes
C Flush the catheter
D Start antibiotics for presumed sepsis
E Stop the patient-controlled analgesic device

29. Steatorrhoea

A 23-year-old woman comes to see you about her stools, which over the last couple of months have become extremely foul smelling, pale in colour and difficult to flush. This has been associated with vague abdominal pains and a bloating sensation. She has found this very embarrassing as she lives in a shared house. She is normally fit and well.

What is the most likely diagnosis?

A Chronic pancreatitis
B Coeliac disease
C Common bile duct obstruction
D Cystic fibrosis
E *Giardia* infection

30. Management of Parkinson's disease (1)

An 83-year-old man who was diagnosed as having Parkinson's disease 3 years ago has been treated with levodopa (L-DOPA). Whilst he initially responded well to therapy, he has started to be increasingly still, and has fallen more in the last 4 months despite no intercurrent illness or change in L-DOPA therapy.

Which is the best management option?

A Add a dopamine agonist (e.g. ropinerole)
B Add a peripheral dopamine antagonist (e.g. domperidone)
C Decrease L-DOPA therapy
D Increase L-DOPA therapy
E Stop L-DOPA therapy

31. Autoantibodies

Which antibody can you expect to see in primary biliary cirrhosis (PBC)?

A ANA
B ANCA
C Anti-mitochondrial antibody
D Anti-phospholipid antibodies
E Anti-smooth muscle antibodies

32. Coronary circulation

The left anterior descending coronary artery usually supplies:

A The anterior wall of the left ventricle and the atrio-ventricular node
B The anterior wall of the left ventricle and the inter-ventricular septum
C The anterior wall of the left ventricle, atrio-ventricular node and the inter-ventricular septum
D The inter-ventricular septum and the inferior part of the left ventricle
E The sino-atrial node, the atrio-ventricular node and the inferior part of the left ventricle

33. Management of anaemia

A 42-year-old woman with menorrhagia is complaining of tiredness. The GP does some blood tests, which reveal hypochromic microcytic anaemia, a decreased ferritin level and a raised total iron binding capacity. Platelets were slightly raised.

Which of the following is the best treatment for this anaemia?

A Erythropoietin
B Iron chelators
C Iron supplementation
D Regular transfusion
E Regular venesection

34. ACE inhibitors

In which of the following circumstances should angiotensin-converting enzyme (ACE) inhibitors be avoided where possible?

A Glomerulonephritis
B Lupus nephritis
C Renal artery stenosis
D Systemic sclerosis with renal involvement
E All of the above

35. Microbiology

Which of the following correctly describes *Staphylococcus aureus*?

A Anaerobic rod
B Gram-negative coccus
C Gram-negative rod
D Gram-positive coccus
E Gram-positive rod

36. Skin lesions (1)

A 78-year-old retired groundskeeper presents with a 2 cm skin lump on his temple. He is unsure how long it has been there. It appears to have a rolled, shiny edge with telangiectasia and a central ulcerated area.

Which of the following is the most likely diagnosis?

A Actinic keratosis
B Basal cell carcinoma
C Keratoacanthoma
D Malignant melanoma
E Squamous cell carcinoma

37. Diagnosis of abdominal pain (1)

A 54-year-old woman presents to the emergency department with a 2-month history of intermittent right upper quadrant pain. The pain is sharp in nature and radiates round to the back. On examination there is no jaundice, no hepatomegaly and she is apyrexial. Liver function tests and an amylase are normal. She has no history of recent foreign travel.

What is the most likely diagnosis?

A Biliary colic
B Cholangitis
C Hepatitis A
D Hepatitis C
E Pancreatitis

38. Ankylosing spondylitis

A 23-year-old man presents with a several-months history of lower back pain and stiffness.

Which of the following symptoms would make you think of ankylosing spondylitis (AS) as the diagnosis?

A Asymmetrical tenderness on palpation over the lumbosacral spine
B HLA-DR4 genotype
C Pain present on waking in the early morning
D Scoliosis present on examination
E Worse after heavy lifting

39. Mitral stenosis

A 75-year-old woman in the pre-assessment clinic tells you she has mitral stenosis.

Which of the following is not a sign of mitral stenosis?

A Bifid P-wave
B Diastolic opening snap heart sound
C Double impulse apex beat
D Mid-diastolic murmur
E Peripheral cyanosis

40. Management of facial weakness

A 35-year-old man presents with a 2-day history of right-sided facial weakness. He is otherwise fit and well. There is no past history of neurological symptoms. There is no history of preceding infection. On examination, the middle ear is normal, the salivary glands are not enlarged, and there are no other cranial nerves affected. The forehead is not spared. Neurological examination of the limbs is unremarkable. Routine investigations are all normal.

Which of the following represents the most reasonable management plan?

A Aspirin, dipyridamole, a statin and an angiotensin-converting enzyme (ACE) inhibitor
B Penicillin-based antibiotic therapy and antiviral therapy
C Steroids
D Steroids and penicillin-based antibiotic therapy
E Steroids, antiviral therapy and eye protection

41. Pathological fracture

A 51-year-old man is found to have a pathological fracture of his femur. Investigations reveal immunoglobulin light chains in the urine.

What is his diagnosis?

A Benign monoclonal gammopathy
B Bone metastases
C Multiple myeloma
D Osteoporosis
E Vitamin D deficiency

42. Management of HIV

A 35-year-old man is diagnosed with human immunodeficiency virus (HIV) infection.

Which of the following indicates that highly active antiretroviral therapy (HAART) should be commenced?

A Fever and weight loss >10 kg
B Viral load >50 copies/ml
C Viral load >100 copies/ml
D CD4 count <200 cells/mm^3
E CD4 count <500 cells/mm^3

43. Tetralogy of Fallot

An anxious mum has read on the internet about tetralogy of Fallot as she is convinced her little boy may have it.

Which of the following does not fit the diagnosis?

A Her child is small for his age
B Her child is cyanotic
C His pulse exhibits a radio-femoral delay
D Her child exhibits a loud systolic murmur
E Her child can relive symptoms just by squatting

44. Investigation of dysphagia

A 45-year-old man presents with intermittent difficulty in swallowing for the last 4 months. This is associated with severe retrosternal pain and regurgitation. He has no risk factors or sinister signs for malignancy.

What is the most important investigation in this case?

A Barium swallow
B Chest X-ray
C CT of the chest
D Endoscopy
E Iron studies

45. Thalassaemia trait

A 55-year-old Asian man with known thalassaemia trait registers with a new GP and is found to have a mild microcytic anaemia on routine testing. He does not complain of any symptoms.

What is the most appropriate treatment?

A Blood transfusion
B Folate supplementation
C Iron chelators
D Iron supplementation
E No treatment required

46. Warfarin therapy

A 72-year-old man is on warfarin for atrial fibrillation. Following a recent chest infection his international normalised ratio (INR) rockets up to 5.2.

What was the most likely cause for this?

A Codeine phosphate
B Erythromycin
C Inappropriate high doses of warfarin
D International normalised ratio (INR) increased in concomitant infection
E Steroid inhalers

47. The painful joint

A 40-year-old man, previously fit and well, limps in to the emergency department with an acutely red, hot, swollen, exquisitely tender knee, which he holds rigid. He is tachycardic and has a temperature of 38.3°C.

Which of the following represents the best approach to diagnosis and management?

A Aspirate a small amount of joint fluid and send it for microscopy under polarised light
B Aspirate a small amount of joint fluid, send the fluid for urgent Gram stain and culture, take blood cultures, and start antibiotics only when you know the sensitivities of any bacteria present
C Aspirate the joint fully, send the fluid for urgent Gram stain and culture, take blood cultures, and start antibiotics only if bacteria are detected on Gram stain of either fluid
D Aspirate the joint fully, send the fluid for urgent Gram stain and culture, take blood cultures, and start antibiotics only when you know sensitivities of any bacteria present
E Aspirate the joint fully, send the fluid for urgent Gram stain and culture, take blood cultures, and start empirical intravenous antibiotics immediately

48. The unresponsive patient (1)

A 29-year-old man is brought to the emergency department having been found unresponsive on a park bench. On examination, his airway is patent and he has a spontaneous respiratory rate of 7, with a saturation rate of 92% on air. There is no abnormality on examination or auscultation of the chest. He has a pulse of 70 bpm and a blood pressure of 110/80 mmHg. The ECG is normal. He has a Glasgow Coma Score (GCS) of 3 and has pinpoint pupils. He has a temperature of 36.8°C and a blood sugar reading of 6. Basic initial management steps include high-flow oxygen administration and intravenous access.

Which of the following might you also implement?

A 500 ml *stat* intravenous fluid challenge
B 50 ml of 50% glucose intravenously *stat*
C Bair hugger
D Flumazenil
E Naloxone

49. Vomiting

A first-time mother comes to visit you with her 10-month-old son. At least once every day her son vomits up his entire feed. The vomiting is not projectile but rather the feed returns to the mouth and spills over his top. She stopped breast-feeding him when he was 6 months old. He is otherwise well in himself, with a normal weight for his age.

What is the most likely diagnosis?

A Gastro-oesophageal reflux disease
B Lactose intolerance
C Physiological posseting
D Pyloric stenosis
E Viral gastroenteritis

50. Weight loss

A 13-year-old girl, who is quiet and withdrawn, comes to see you with her mother. She has a 4-month history of weight loss and secondary amenorrhoea. She has no bowel symptoms. Her body mass index is 16. Apart from being very thin, the examination is otherwise normal. All blood results, including hormone assays, are normal.

What is the most likely diagnosis?

A Anorexia nervosa
B Coeliac disease
C Crohn's disease
D Epstein–Barr virus infection
E Irritable bowel syndrome

Practice Paper 1: Answers

1. Acute coronary syndrome (1)

B. Give 75 mg aspirin *stat*

A *stat* dose of 300 mg aspirin is the correct figure. Low-dose (75 mg) aspirin is used for long-term prevention. ACS is the title given to a collection of cardiac diseases that all share the same atherosclerotic aetiology. ST-elevated MI, non-ST-elevated MI and unstable angina are all caused by stenosed coronary arteries starving the myocardium of oxygen (angina), leading to hypoxic cell death (myocardial infarction). Unstable angina occurs on the cusp of these phenomena, when a rest is no longer adequate to replenish the myocardium with oxygen. Acute coronary stenoses are usually caused by intimal plaque rupture leading to an intraluminal thrombus. Aspirin, clopidogrel and heparin aim to prevent platelets binding and therefore to arrest thrombus growth and dissolve the thrombus. Aspirin can cause stomach ulcers and so, in order to balance risks and benefits, low-dose aspirin is given long term; a higher dose (300 mg) is given acutely. Statins prophylactically lower serum cholesterol, and so it is thought to reduce plaque formation in the first place. ACE inhibitors and beta-blockers reduce afterload and heart rate, so the heart does not have to work as hard – this lowers its oxygen demand, hopefully enough to prevent hypoxic damage.

2. Obstructive renal impairment

E. Systemic sclerosis

Benign prostatic hypertrophy can cause urinary retention and increased pressure in the urinary outflow tract, and as this disease affects older men, who can be quite reluctant to seek help with non-urgent medical problems, this can get to the stage at which kidney function is impaired. Recurrent kidney stones passing into the ureter can cause scarring, especially at narrow sites such as the vesicoureteric junction. Retroperitoneal fibrosis typically involves a fibrosing inflammatory reaction starting in the wall of the aorta and spreading retroperitoneally. The ureters can become embroiled in the fibrous tissue. Obstruction is believed to be due to a loss of peristalsis rather than occlusion. Schistosomiasis is common in the Middle East and parts of Africa, featuring granulomas forming around the eggs of schistosomes in the urinary tract, and these can obstruct the urinary tract. Systemic sclerosis leads to a fibrinoid thickening of the afferent arterioles, leading to reduced renal perfusion and thus renal impairment, but it does not cause an obstructive uropathy.

3. Management of skin lesions (1)

A. Cryotherapy

This man has a past history of likely excessive sun exposure and thus is at risk for sun-related skin disease. This lesion appears to be an actinic keratosis – it is not pigmented (effectively ruling out melanoma), and it is flat rather than raised, making basal cell and squamous cell carcinomata unlikely (although there can be superficial basal cell carcinomas, which are well demarcated and deep red, with less scale). A small mildly erythematous patch with keratotic hypertrophy (scales and horns) is most likely an actinic keratosis (or solar keratosis). Treatment of isolated small lesions is by cryotherapy. It has no concerning features to suggest that excision or histopathological examination is required. Large areas of skin with multiple actinic keratoses can be treated with 5-fluorouracil cream to avoid excessive scarring from cryotherapy, and can be more effective at slowing re-growth.

4. Chest X-ray

A. Trachea deviated to the right, dull to percussion of RUZ, reduced breath sounds on auscultation

A lung collapse would tend to pull the trachea towards the affected side. There would be reduced breath sounds (with or without crackles and bronchial breathing) and dullness to percussion on the affected side.

5. Headaches

D. Polycythaemia rubra vera

Polycythaemia rubra vera is a myeloproliferative disorder characterised by a raised haemoglobin level, red cell count and packed cell volume (haematocrit). The condition is caused by the mutation of a single pluripotent stem cell, which results in the excessive production of erythrocytes and, to a lesser degree, platelets and neutrophils. As a result, the blood becomes extremely viscous causing an increased risk of arterial and venous thrombosis and paradoxical bleeding. Patients often complain of headaches, visual disturbance, lethargy and pruritis that is classically worse after bathing in warm water. Treatment of the polycythaemia rubra vera involves venesection (blood-letting) and chemotherapy with hydroxyurea. If treated appropriately patients tend to survive for many years and often die from non-related causes. Approximately

30% of patients will develop myelofibrosis and 5% will develop acute myeloid leukaemia as part of the disease's natural history.

Secondary polycythaemia is usually caused by the increased secretion of erythropoietin as part of the physiological response to hypoxia in conditions such as chronic obstructive airways disease and cyanotic heart disease. Less frequently erythropoetin is secreted ectopically from tumour cells (e.g. renal cell carcinomas). Occasionally the condition is iatrogenic, caused by the overuse of artificial erythropoietin used in the treatment of conditions such as anaemia of chronic renal failure. Investigating polycythaemia involves referral to a haematologist, who will accurately assess the red cell mass and exclude secondary causes. Bone marrow analysis may be required to diagnose genetic abnormalities. The treatment of secondary polycythaemia involves managing the underlying disease and symptomatic venesection.

Polycythaemia, from Greek *poly* = many + *kytos* = cell

Rubra vera, from Latin *rubra* = red + *vera* = true

6. Chronic obstructive pulmonary disease

B. Inhaled corticosteroids

Smoking cessation is important in patients with chronic obstructive pulmonary disease and it is the only intervention proven to decelerate the decline in FEV_1. Pneumococcal and annual influenza vaccination is provided to reduce the risk of exacerbation of chronic obstructive pulmonary disease (COPD) by viral infection. Short-acting bronchodilators (e.g. β2 agonists or anticholinergics) help in reducing breathlessness and exercise limitation. A combined therapy of these two bronchodilators is used if the patient is still symptomatic with just one type of inhaled bronchodilator. A long-acting bronchodilator is added if symptoms persist with the combined therapy. Inhaled corticosteroids are added if FEV_1<50% and the patient has two or more exacerbations in a 12-month period.

7. Management of asthma (1)

D. Leukotriene receptor antagonists

The altered level of consciousness, exhaustion, silent chest, PaO_2 <8.0 kPa, and "normal $PaCO_2$" 4.6–6.0 kPa all suggest that this patient has life-threatening asthma. High-flow oxygen is needed to maintain a saturation level of 94–98%. In acute life-threatening asthma, the nebulised route (oxygen driven) is recommended. Steroids reduce mortality, relapses, subsequent hospital admission and requirement for beta-2 agonist therapy. Magnesium sulphate has bronchodilation effects and is used in acute severe asthma if there is not a good initial response to inhaled bronchodilator therapy, and also in life-threatening asthma. There is insufficient evidence at present to show that leukotriene receptor antagonists are effective in the management of acute asthma.

8. Collapse (1)

B. Hypertrophic obstructive cardiomyopathy (HOCM)

HOCM is a congenital disease of the myocardium. The left ventricular myocardium becomes so thick that the outflow tract becomes restricted. This restriction is mechanically exacerbated by the muscular systolic contraction generated by vigorous exercise, hence, hard exercise leads to a fall off in output, which leads to syncope. Sufferers are vulnerable to sudden death, of which there may be a family history as the disease is inherited (autosomal dominant).

9. Eczema versus psoriasis

C. Localised to flexures rather than extensors

Whilst nail pitting and ridging may occasionally be seen with eczema, nail changes are much more commonly associated with psoriasis, usually with nail pitting and onycholysis (detachment of parts of the nail from the nail bed), and occasionally with subungual hyperkeratosis (extensive keratotic growth beneath the nail). Distal interphalangeal joint disease (in this case with pain and swelling) is one of five characteristic patterns of 'psoriatic arthropathy', which overall around 5–10% of those with psoriasis will develop at some stage – in some cases, before the outbreak of psoriasis. The five patterns are distal interphalangeal arthritis, symmetrical polyarthritis, asymmetrical oligoarthritis, spondyloarthropathy and arthritis mutilans, which is a severe destructive arthropathy mainly affecting the hands. Eczema is more commonly localised to flexures, whereas psoriatic plaques are more typically localised to extensor surfaces. That said, there is a variety of psoriasis that more often develops later in life, in which the plaques appear in well-opposed flexural surfaces such as the groin and submammary area. Psoriasis more often presents with well-demarcated lesions or "plaques", whereas eczematous lesions more often are described as "patches". Psoriasis typically responds well to sunlight and thus would be worse in the winter months. This is the basis of ultraviolet (UV) therapy for psoriasis, and patients may be advised to expose affected skin (within reason) to sunshine where possible – although this is often difficult due to cosmetic concerns.

10. Diagnosis of multiple sclerosis (1)

D. Periventricular white matter lesions not necessarily matching the clinical picture

Longitudinally extensive transverse myelitis is unusual in multiple sclerosis (MS), and is more typical of neuromyelitis optica (NMO or Devic disease), a rare autoimmune central nervous system demyelinating disease affecting the spinal cord and optic nerves. Once thought to be a subtype of MS, however, it is now known to be a distinct disease strongly associated with anti-aquaporin 4 antibodies. Whilst grey matter is affected in MS, and there is some evidence that overall grey matter volume decreases in MS and correlates with disability, focal grey matter inflammatory lesions would not be expected, and the focal lesions are in fact found in the white matter. The cerebellum and brainstem are affected in multiple sclerosis, however, not exclusively. White matter lesions are classically described as "periventricular", and the lesions found do not always correlate with a clinical focus of disease. This is because the central nervous system (CNS) inflammation does not always cause demyelination or axonal damage of clinical significance, and the CNS can recover from these foci of inflammation.

Eugene Devic, French neurologist (1858-1930)

11. The multidisciplinary team

A. District nurse

District nurses provide care within the community. Their workload includes looking after house-bound and recently discharged patients, helping them manage wound dressings and monitor medications.

Social workers look after the individuals and their contacts from a social perspective (e.g. families, friends). They also liaise with other organisations including schools, the National Health Service (NHS), housing agencies and charitable organisations to plan packages of care and support for the individual. The health visitor (a qualified nurse) takes over care of a newborn from community midwives after the first 10 days of birth. Health visitors also run health promotion and smoking cessation clinics. An orthotist is someone who measures, designs and fits orthoses (an external device that can be applied to correct a deformity, rather like a splint).

Orthotics, from Greek *ortho* = straighten

12. Diagnosis of chest pain (1)

E. I'm not sure, we need to do more tests

This man has left bundle branch block (LBBB). The ST elevation does not therefore confirm MI as the ST elevation could be due to the abnormal left ventricular depolarisation. If the clinical features are in keeping, he could be treated for a presumed myocardial infarction until 12-hour troponin blood test results are available to confirm or deny the diagnosis and/or other ECG changes appear, such as pronounced Q-waves growing over time. Bundle branch block can be remembered by: WiLLiaM and MaRRoW. LBBB (the "L"s in WiLLiaM) is reported by a broad S-wave (or deep Q- and S-waves) in the right-hand leads (forming a "W" in the QRS of V1–3, mainly V1) and a pair of R-waves in the left-hand leads (forming an "M" in the QRS of V4–6, mainly V6). Either way, the QRS complexes will be broad, even if the "W"s and "M"s are not obvious. Right bundle branch block (RBBB) reports the reverse: an "M" in the QRS of leads V1–3 and a "W" in the QRS of V4–6.

Other causes of a LBBB include aortic stenosis, dilated cardiomyopathy, chronic hypertension and extensive coronary artery disease without MI. The finding of LBBB is always pathological. New LBBB with typical features is consistent with the diagnosis of an acute coronary syndrome.

13. Risk factors for ischaemic heart disease

E. 12 U/week of alcohol

Moderate alcohol consumption can reduce coronary artery disease but heavy drinking increases it. All the other options increase the risk of ischaemic heart disease and are modifiable.

14. Diagnosis of cough (1)

C. *Legionella pneumophila*

Legionella pneumophila tends to colonise in water tanks kept at below 60°C (e.g. hotel air-conditioning and hot water systems). Patients who acquire *Legionella pneumophila* infection will present with non-specific symptoms such as fever, myalgia, headache, confusion and diarrhoea. Blood tests reveal hyponatraemia, abnormal liver function tests (elevated liver enzymes, hypoalbuminaemia) and an elevated creatine kinase. The diagnosis is confirmed by *Legionella* serology or urine *Legionella* antigen.

15. Diagnosis of vertigo

B. Delayed onset (a few seconds) torsional nystagmus on descent facing one side only

Benign paroxysmal positional vertigo (BPPV) is caused by debris blocking the normal flow of endolymph in the labyrinth, leading to misreporting of positional change by the vestibules, and a discrepancy between actual position and the position of the head according to the vestibules. Thus, nystagmus occurs as two different inputs compete for different oculomotor outputs, and vertigo (the perception that the world is moving) ensues. This happens only when the head moves and there is no vertigo with a still head. It usually affects one side only, and thus Hallpike's manoeuvre (below) only reveals nystagmus when the patient's head is tilted back whilst they face one side and not the other. Torsional nystagmus is normally seen after a few seconds of the head being tilted back – it is important to keep the patient lying back for some time. The nystagmus should wear off after around 20 seconds, and on repeat testing it lasts a shorter amount of time ("fatiguing"). This is the basis of vestibular exercises, which are designed so that compensatory mechanisms may be induced more swiftly and the vertigo attacks will thus become less frequent and less disabling.

The Hallpike test is conducted as follows:

1. The patient sits upright with their legs extended.
2. The patient's head is then rotated 45 degrees.
3. The patient is then made to lie down quickly and the head is held in extension.
4. The patient's eyes are then observed. A positive test will result in nystagmus towards the affected side after a 5–10 second latent period.

The Epley manoeuvre effectively treats most cases of BPPV. In this manoeuvre:

1. The patient sits upright with their legs extended.
2. The patient's head is rotated towards the affected side.
3. With the head still turned, the patient is laid flat past the horizontal (as in the Hallpike test). This position is held for 30 seconds.
4. The patient's head is then turned to the opposite side in the reclined position (and held for 30 seconds).
5. The patient is now rolled onto their side (the side opposite to the affected ear) with the head still turned for 30 seconds.
6. The patient is then made to sit upright, still with the head turned to the opposite side of the lesion (for 30 seconds).
7. The patient's head is turned back to the midline with the neck flexed 45 degrees (for 30 seconds).

Charles Skinner Hallpike, English otologist (1900-1979)

16. Epistaxis

E. Wegener granulomatosis

Wegener granulomatosis is characterised by systemic vasculitis that involves small and medium vessels. The classic triad consists of upper and lower respiratory tract involvement and pauci-immune glomerulonephritis. The upper respiratory tract involvement includes otorrhoea, sinusitis, nasal discharge and crusting, epistaxis, oral and nasal ulcers, mucosal bleeding and inflammation, nasal septal perforation and a saddle nose deformity. The lower respiratory tract involvement includes cough, haemoptysis, chest pain and shortness of breath. Microscopic haematuria is a common finding in Wegener granulomatosis. A positive ANCA test in the setting of this classic triad is sufficient to diagnose Wegener granulomatosis without a histological confirmation. Goodpasture syndrome is caused by an anti-glomerular basement membrane antibody that results in pulmonary haemorrhage and glomerulonephritis without involvement of the upper respiratory tract.

Friedrich Wegener, German pathologist (1907-1990)

17. Diarrhoea (1)

B. *Clostridium difficile* infection

C. difficile is a major cause of antibiotic-association diarrhoea and hospital morbidity within the country. *C. difficile* is a Gram-positive commensal bacterium of the gastrointestinal tract that can proliferate when the intestinal flora is disturbed by the use of broad-spectrum antibiotics. Third-generation cephalosporins were particularly implicated with this and their use is not advised in the over 65s. *C. difficile* produces two enterotoxins (A and B) that cause severe inflammation of the intestinal mucosa and the formation of thick fibrous bands (pseudomembranes) in the intestine, which can harbour large numbers of bacteria. The patient often has significant diarrhoea (with or without blood), which can lead to rapid dehydration, electrolyte imbalance and death. *C. difficile* is treated by managing the patient's fluid and electrolyte balance and prescribing a course of metronidazole or vancomycin. Much effort is being placed in the prevention of *Clostridium* infection by promoting the correct use of broad-spectrum antibiotics and educating staff and visitors regarding the importance of hand washing. It should be noted that the spores of *C. difficile* are not destroycd by alcohol hand gel, meaning that soap and water must be used every time!

Clostridium, from Latin *kloster* = spindle (shape)

Difficile, from Latin *difficile* = difficult

18. Diagnosis of malaria

E. Three thick and thin blood films on consecutive days

Falciparum antigen dipstick testing is a useful, cheap and labour-unintensive way to diagnose or exclude falciparum malaria, however, a well-examined blood film is far more sensitive. Thick and thin blood films are done because thick films make pickup of low-level parasitaemias more likely and thin blood films allow species identification and quantification (more than 2%

of red blood cells being parasitised is a prognostic marker of severe disease). Blood films should be taken on 3 consecutive days, as an initial film may be negative due to the lifecycle of the parasite. Blood cultures should be taken as there may be coexisting bacteraemia ("algid malaria"), however they do not grow *Plasmodium* species. Liver biopsy is not used to investigate malaria.

19. Electrocardiogram (1)

A. First-degree heart block

Analyse an ECG methodically. Start with rate: bradycardia if less than 60/ min, tachycardic if greater than 100/min. Next, check the rhythm is regular; this can be trickier than it seems, especially if the patient is tachycardic. The axis is determined by looking at the amplitude of the QRS complex relative to lead II, i.e. lead II is 0°, lead I is −45° and lead III is +135°. If the QRS amplitude is greatest in lead II and leads I and III have identical, lesser magnitudes, then the QRS is not deviated. If it is most positive in lead I, then it is deviated to the left. If it is most positive in lead III, then it is deviated to the right. Remember that the QRS complex is the charge "washing" through the myocardium. The axis of the QRS helps us to visualise the comparative muscularity of the right and left ventricles, which may in turn highlight a disease process against which a given ventricle is fighting, e.g. aortic stenosis leading to left ventricular hypertrophy resulting in left axis deviation. An axis outside of ±30 degrees can be said to be deviated. The P-wave position and shape should be noted. The PR interval should be less than 0.20 seconds. In this case, there is a fixed delay (through the atrio-ventricular node) which is called first-degree heart block. QRS amplitude, shape and duration are all significant. A width >3 small squares (at 25 mm/s ECG speed) is equivalent to 0.12 seconds, and this is the boundary between QRS complexes being narrow or broad. Ventricular tachycardias are broad (and faster than 90/ min). A broad complex may well contain a distortion in shape in one of the leads indicating bundle branch block. This ECG has a narrow QRS complex. Finally, the T-wave size and the QT duration should be observed. It is always good practice to compare a current ECG to a previous ECG but this should not prevent you reviewing and summarising the ECG. If there is any doubt, and no old ECGs are available, a repeat test can be requested.

20. Investigation of deranged liver function tests

A. Alpha-1-antitrypsin serum levels

Alpha-1 antitrypsin (A1AT) deficiency is an autosomal recessive disorder. About 1% of COPD patients will have this genetic abnormality. A1AT is a serine protease inhibitor normally synthesised in the liver whose role is to cleave and inhibit the proteolytic enzyme neutrophil elastase. Absence of A1AT leads to pulmonary emphysema and liver disease in some patients.

The gene is located on chromosome 14 and there are variants that correlate to disease severity and presentation. The most severe forms can present with cirrhosis in childhood. Treatment is supportive.

21. Epigastric pain (1)

A. Acute pericarditis

The ECG shows widespread saddle-shaped ST elevation, a typical change associated with acute pericarditis. Viral pericarditis can be caused by a preceding viral respiratory tract infection; bilateral pulmonary effusions may also be present. Pleurisy – inflammation of the pleura – does not directly cause ECG changes and does not correlate as well with the sign of postural pain changes. Myocardial infarction and angina are unlikely to cause pain of this nature, but a 12-hour troponin test should be requested. A painful pulmonary embolism would usually affect the oxygen saturations and not necessarily provide ECG evidence. If in doubt, blood gas testing should be undertaken.

22. Gout prophylaxis

C. Start allopurinol at least 2 weeks after the acute attack has settled with NSAID cover and increase until his urate level is below 300 µmol/L

Long-term diclofenac carries the risk of side effects such as peptic ulceration and renal impairment, and will achieve nothing between attacks as there is no inflammation. Similarly, depot steroid injections may be used in acute attacks but long-term steroids carry the risk of immunosuppression as well as many other side effects. The underlying pathology in gout is hyperuricaemia, therefore prophylactic treatment should aim to reduce serum urate. Allopurinol inhibits xanthine oxidase, which produces urate, and thus lowers serum urate. It can precipitate acute attacks and therefore should not be used within 2–4 weeks of an acute attack, and should be started with either NSAIDs or colchicine used at least 2 weeks before and 4 weeks after starting. Long-term colchicine is not recommended for prophylaxis. Sulfinpyrazone is a second-line prophylactic agent.

23. Hepatomegaly

A. End-stage cirrhosis

Hepatomegaly describes the enlargement of the liver. It is detected clinically by palpating the right upper quadrant during inspiration. As the patient inspires the liver is displaced inferiorly by the lungs onto the examiner's hand. In normal individuals the liver should not be palpated with the exception of children and particularly thin patients. The presence of hepatomegaly is usually described in terms of size, e.g. number of finger-breadths below the costal margin. The texture of the liver edge should also be documented and it should be noted whether it is smooth or craggy. Conditions that cause hepatomegaly with a smooth margin include viral hepatitis, biliary tract obstruction, hepatic vein thrombosis (Budd–Chiari syndrome), right heart failure and myeloproliferative disease. Hepatomegaly with a craggy border is usually associated with hepatic metastatic disease and polycystic disease.

End-stage cirrhosis does not result in hepatomegaly. Early liver damage often causes hepatomegaly and fatty infiltration, but as the damage progresses and fibrosis ensues, replacing the normal tissue architecture, the liver becomes small and scarred.

24. Sclerosing cholangitis

E. Ulcerative colitis (UC)

Sclerosing cholangitis is a condition causing inflammation, fibrosis and subsequent stricture formation of the bile ducts, leading to cholestasis and eventual cirrhosis. These changes occur in the intra- and extrahepatic bile ducts. There is a strong association with inflammatory bowel disease, most commonly ulcerative colitis, with about 80% of patients with sclerosing cholangitis having coexistent disease (note that although only ~5% of patients with UC have concomitant sclerosing cholangitis). These patients present with the effects of jaundice. Liver biopsy is diagnostic. Treatment is primarily symptomatic. Ursodeoxycholic acid may delay disease progression and liver transplant is curative in some cases. Purely extrahepatic disease may be surgically treated.

25. Investigation of status epilepticus

E. Phenytoin levels

There are many reasons why this man may be in status epilepticus, but the most common cause, and a quick and simple one to rule out, would be low antiepileptic drug levels. This is estimated to be the cause of around 30% of status episodes. Alcoholism is prevalent amongst the homeless population, and many antiepileptics are metabolised by the cytochrome p450 system in the liver (phenytoin included). Chronic alcohol abuse can induce increased cytochrome p450 activity, which could then lower the phenytoin levels. His compliance with phenytoin therapy could be poor given his social situation. Regarding the other investigations, brain imaging will be poor or impossible as he is still fitting, and EEG is only indicated if he is still fitting after various management steps have been undertaken and he is taken to the intensive treatment unit (ITU) for general anaesthesia. Regarding the echocardiogram, the homeless population is indeed at risk of endocarditis, which could lead to subsequent septic embolisation to the brain, causing the seizures. A murmur is also heard, however this would be a less likely cause than low phenytoin levels, and less easy to treat acutely if found. Magnetic resonance imaging (MRI) of the head should be carried out beforehand if an intracranial cause such as septic emboli is being considered. Furthermore, regarding the possibly new murmur and fever, the fever could be due to the seizure activity, and the murmur could be benign or old (it may be worth contacting the GP or searching for the patient's old hospital notes to see if it has been investigated).

26. Shortness of breath (1)

B. Mitral stenosis

A history of recurrent rheumatic fever would reinforce this diagnosis. This patient's mitral valve is restricting the onward flow of freshly oxygenated blood from the lungs. This back-pressure is the cause of his pulmonary oedema (inspiratory crackles, frothy pinky–white sputum). The loud first heart sound is due to the mitral valve leaflets shutting abruptly at the start of systole, as if a door ajar were closed with the same force as a door wide open. The mid-diastolic murmur is the turbulent flow of blood through the restricted opening. It is low-frequency and so is best heard with the bell of the stethoscope. A malar flush may be visible upon the face of the patient.

Rheumatic fever is predominantly a disease of the developing world, and is usually seen in children between 5 and 15 years of age. The condition develops 2–4 weeks after a group A beta-haemolytic streptococcal pharyngitis. In susceptible individuals, the antibodies formed against the bacterial carbohydrate cell wall cross-react with antigens in the heart, joints and skin in a process known as molecular mimicry. The immune response in the heart causes myocarditis, pericarditis and endocarditis, resulting in valve destruction, conduction defects, arrhythmia and congestive cardiac failure.

The diagnosis of rheumatic fever is made using the modified Duckett Jones criteria, requiring either two major criteria OR one major and two minor criteria PLUS evidence of streptococcal infection (e.g. anti-streptolysin-O titres):

Modified Duckett Jones criteria

Major
      Pancarditis
      Polyarthritis
      Sydenham chorea (St Vitus' dance)
      Erythema marginatum
      Subcutaneous nodules

Minor
>   Fever
>   Arthralgia
>   High erythrocyte sedimentation rate or white cell count
>   Heart block

Chorea, from Latin *chorea* = dance

Saint Vitus' dance (*chorea sancti viti* in Latin) was a mediaeval festival that celebrated Vitus, the patron saint of dancers, actors and comedians

T Duckett Jones, American physician (1899-1954)

27. Aortic regurgitation

E. Systemic lupus erythematosus (SLE)

SLE can cause myocarditis, pericarditis and endocarditis. Whilst the latter manifestation can cause valvular vegetations, they are rarely symptomatic and are more likely to be diagnosed post mortem. Causes of aortic regurgitation, which presents primarily as dyspnoea, include idiopathic aortic root dilatation, syphilitic aortitis, aortic dissection and rheumatic fever. It is also associated with ankylosing spondylosis and Marfan syndrome. In addition to a collapsing pulse, aortic regurgitation also presents with an early diastolic murmur, a mid-diastolic rumble (Austin Flint murmur), de Musset's sign (synchronous head nodding), Quincke's sign (pulsing nail bed), Traube's sign ("pistol shot" sound at the femoral artery as its walls slacken and then crack taught like a sail in the wind) and a laterally displaced apex beat.

Austin Flint, American physician (1812-1886)

Alfred de Musset, French novelist who died from aortic regurgitation. His brother noticed his head used to bob with his pulse

Heinrich Irenaeus Quincke, German physician (1842-1922)

Ludwig Traube, German physician (1818-1876)

28. Management of oliguria (1)

B. Fluid challenge of 500 ml normal saline over 10 minutes

It is likely that there has been a fair bit of blood loss intraoperatively. The operation notes could be checked to confirm this. It is major orthopaedic surgery and she has conjunctival pallor, which make it seem fairly likely. She seems clinically dry with tachycardia, reduced blood pressure and delayed capillary refill, which follows on from the intraoperative blood loss with slow intravenous fluid replacement (12 hourly). She could also theoretically be septic, but low-grade pyrexia is common postoperatively and there is no presumed source. A urine dip test could be taken to rule out urine infection. Hypovolaemia is more parsimonious. She does not have heart failure and should be able to tolerate a fluid challenge; this is a quick way to find out whether hypovolaemia was to blame. Normal saline should be used rather than 5% dextrose, as the saline will remain largely intravascular, whereas the 5% dextrose, after rapid metabolism of the dextrose, is essentially water, and this will enter the tissues and not increase the intravascular volume as much. Intravenous fluids could then subsequently be sped up. Flushing the catheter can rule out obstruction of the catheter, but the bladder was not palpable on examination and there was no previous bleeding to suggest potential obstruction; this is quick and does not harm the patient so could also be tried. Morphine does not commonly reduce urine output or lead to renal failure. It can cause urinary retention, however a catheter is *in situ* so this is not the cause here.

29. Steatorrhoea

B. Coeliac disease

The description of this woman's stools is classical for steatorrhoea, which is a malabsorption of fat from the diet. There are many causes for this including all of the above. However, coeliac disease is the most likely diagnosis in a woman of this age group with no other symptoms of respiratory distress or foreign travel. If the diagnosis is in doubt then repeated stool specimens should be sent for *Giardia* cysts and ova identification.

30. Management of Parkinson's disease (1)

A. Add a dopamine agonist (e.g. ropinerole)

The general theory of Parkinson's disease management is that early on, when there are still many SNpc neurons surviving, L-DOPA is more useful as this precursor then increases the amount of dopamine being released in a physiological manner to allow movement. However, as the disease progresses and the SNpc neurons reduce in number, L-DOPA increases will not be able to increase the functional amount of dopamine being released in the basal ganglia and so dopamine agonists should increasingly be used. This is less physiological but improves bradykinesia. At the latter stage, increasing L-DOPA is unlikely to provide a benefit; decreasing L-DOPA may be advisable but not without a dopamine agonist, and stopping it altogether is likely to worsen function. The addition of a dopamine agonist may relieve bradykinesia and postural instability at this stage. A peripheral dopamine antagonist: 1) will not act centrally and 2) would exacerbate symptoms, so would be no help. Domperidone can in fact be used to relieve medication-associated nausea in Parkinson disease.

31. Autoantibodies

C. Anti-mitochondrial antibody

PBC is a rare condition predominantly affecting women in their 50s. The aetiology is thought to be autoimmune. There is chronic granulomatous inflammation of the interlobular bile ducts causing cholestasis. Presentation is through the effects of cholestasis – jaundice, pruritis, hepatomegaly and pain. It may also be picked up early by deranged liver function tests in the asymptomatic patient. Diagnosis is made by liver biopsy, and anti-mitochondrial antibodies may be present. Management is threefold: 1) symptomatic to reduce itchiness and prevent osteoporosis, 2) specific medications to improve absorption and finally 3) disease-modifying drugs such as ursodeoxycholic acid (which reduces cholestasis). Recent evidence however suggests that ursodeoxycholic acid does not improve mortality. Liver transplant may be an option in some candidates with end-stage disease.

32. Coronary circulation

B. The anterior wall of the left ventricle and the inter-ventricular septum

The left anterior descending artery normally supplies the anterior wall of the left ventricle and the inter-ventricular septum. It arises from the left coronary artery, as does the circumflex artery, which supplies the posterior and lateral sides of the left ventricle. The right coronary artery usually supplies the sino-atrial node, atrio-ventricular node, right ventricle and inferior part of the left ventricle.

33. Management of anaemia

C. Iron supplementation

These blood tests reveal iron-deficiency anaemia, which is most commonly treated with oral iron supplementation.

Iron deficiency anaemia (IDA) is defined as a haemoglobin concentration below 13.5 g/dL in males or 11.5 g/dL in females, in association with a low mean cell volume (MCV) and evidence of depleted iron stores (i.e. a low ferritin and a raised total iron binding capacity). In the developed world IDA is usually secondary to chronic blood loss from gastrointestinal, uterine and urinary tract sources. (Worldwide, hookworm infection and schistosomiasis are common causes.) In cases where the source of bleeding is obvious, further investigation is usually not necessary and treatment can begin; however in many instances bleeding goes unnoticed and is secondary to a more sinister cause such as gastrointestinal malignancy. As such, patients with IDA without an obvious cause must be referred for investigation of the upper and lower gastrointestinal tract in the first instance.

To treat IDA the underlying cause must be corrected and iron stores replenished. The most appropriate method of replacing iron is with oral supplementation (e.g. ferrous sulphate 200 mg tds). Haemoglobin should rise by 1 g/dL every 7 days. Treatment is given until haemoglobin concentrations return to normal and for a further 3–6 months in order to replenish the depleted iron stores. If the haemoglobin fails to respond as expected you must consider non-compliance/concordance with treatment, malabsorption and misdiagnosis. Intramuscular and intravenous preparations of iron do exist but are usually reserved for cases of refractory anaemia secondary to malabsorption and chronic disease. Blood transfusion should only be considered in severe and symptomatic anaemia (e.g. Hb <8 g/dL). Expect the haemoglobin concentration to increase by 1 g/dL per unit of red blood cells given.

34. ACE inhibitors

C. Renal artery stenosis

Glomerulonephritis and lupus nephritis are both autoimmune in origin and aside from supportive measures and renoprotection with drugs including ACE inhibitors, immunosuppression is commonly used and works with varying effect. Systemic sclerosis can affect the afferent arterioles with fibrinoid thickening and vessel narrowing, which can come on rapidly ("scleroderma renal crisis"). Immunosuppression is often unhelpful, whereas ACE inhibitors are of immense benefit and can halt progression of loss of renal function and sometimes even partially reverse it. In severe renal artery stenosis, ACE inhibitors can further reduce or abolish glomerular filtration. This is because angiotensin normally increases glomerular capillary perfusion pressure, and so when ACE inhibitors reduce this ability, with a background of already grossly reduced renal perfusion, the glomerular filtration rate will fall. For this reason, the response to ACE inhibitors should be monitored in patients with renal failure (and especially so in patients with known peripheral arterial disease), and if renal function worsens, various imaging techniques can be used to look for renal artery stenosis (such as Doppler ultrasound and renal arteriography). Overall, whilst ACE inhibitors should be avoided where possible in patients with renal artery stenosis, they are beneficial in protecting the kidneys of renal failure patients, and under specialist supervision can be started at a reduced dose in patients with renal artery stenosis, especially if there is hypertension that cannot be controlled by other means.

35. Microbiology

D. Gram-positive coccus

Staphylococcus aureus is a facultative anaerobe, i.e. it can survive without using oxygen in its metabolism but will make use of it when available.

Gram-negative cocci include *Neisseria gonorrhoea* and *Neisseria meningitides*. Gram-negative rods include *Escherichia coli*, *Salmonella* species, *Haemophilus influenzae*, *Pseudomonas aeruginosa*, *Enterobacter* species and *Helicobacter pylori*. Gram-positive rods include *Clostridium* species and *Listeria*, whereas Gram-positive cocci of human significance are either *Staphylococci* or *Streptococci*. Many *Staphylococci* are skin flora in humans and commonly cause cellulitis and intravenous line and wound infections. Initial appearance of bacteria upon Gram staining (positive or negative, cocci or rods) can, together with the clinical picture, suggest likely organisms and guide empirical antibiotic therapies before culture and sensitivities have been performed.

Staphylococcus, from Greek staphyle = bunch of grapes (reference to the clumping of cocci)

36. Skin lesions (1)

B. Basal cell carcinoma

The rolled edge, pearly appearance and telangiectasia are all classic features of basal cell carcinoma. The history of sun exposure creates concerns of skin cancer. It is not described as melanocytic, therefore malignant melanoma seems highly unlikely (although amelanocytic malignant melanomas exist). Squamous cell carcinomas are ill-defined keratotic nodules that often ulcerate more so than basal cell carcinomas (BCCs). They can grow faster than the slow growing BCCs. The risk factors are largely the same, however, and the combined investigation and management of both is simple: excise and send for histology (usually curative and diagnostic). Keratoacanthomas are rapidly growing benign tumours that often mimic squamous cell carcinomas. They can become quite large and typically develop a central ulceration and necrosis pattern. They should be excised to exclude squamous cell carcinoma as it is difficult to tell the two apart, although many resolve spontaneously. Actinic keratoses are small erythematous silver-scaled patches or papules that are common in sun damage, but are benign and can be treated (if sufficiently large to warrant treatment) by cryotherapy, or if diffuse can be treated by topical 5-fluorouracil cream or imiquimod cream (to save repeated cryotherapy and associated minor scarring). They have the potential to turn into squamous cell carcinomas after several years.

37. Diagnosis of abdominal pain (1)

A. Biliary colic

Biliary colic is a localised inflammation of the gallbladder due to gallstones. The name in itself is a misnomer as the pain is rarely "colicky" in nature, but more likely to be a severe and constant pain that may be related to the ingestion of fatty foods. Gallstones typically present in patients with the 5 Fs – fat, forty, female, fair (Caucasian) and fertile (pre-menopausal). Management is by removal of the gallbladder (cholecystectomy), usually performed laparoscopically.

38. Ankylosing spondylitis

C. Pain present on waking in the early morning

AS is an inflammatory disorder of the back that is more common in males. Patients present with lower back pain and stiffness of insidious onset that is worse in the morning and gets better with exercise. There is poor spinal flexion and in severe cases patients develop a rigid lower spine with a hunch (known as the "question mark posture" or "hang dog posture"). AS may also affect the large joints asymmetrically (although it affects the lumbar joints symmetrically). AS is associated with a number of extra-articular features that are remembered by the five As: Apical lung fibrosis, Anterior uveitis, Achilles tendonitis/plantar fasciitis, Aortic regurgitation, and Amyloidosis.

This diagnosis of AS is made using Schober's test: two fingers are placed 10 cm apart on the lower back of the patient (5 cm above and below the L5 vertebra in the midline) and the patient is asked to flex. An increase between the fingers of <5 cm indicates spinal stiffness. X-ray of the hip shows blurred margins of the sacroiliac joints (sacroiliitis). Characteristic radiological features of the spine in AS include erosion of the corners of the vertebral bodies (Romanus lesions), the development of bony spurs (syndesmophytes) and calcification of the spinal ligaments (bamboo spine). Treatment options in AS are physiotherapy, exercise and slow-release non-steroidal anti-inflammatory drugs (NSAIDs), e.g. indomethacin. Most patients manage to lead a normal life, although severe cases may impair ventilation.

AS is an example of a seronegative spondyloarthropathy – diseases associated with HLA-B27 that are characterised by a lack of rheumatoid factor (hence "seronegative"). Other spondyloarthropathies are psoriatic arthritis, Reiter disease and enteropathic arthritis. The HLA-DR4 genotype is associated with rheumatoid arthritis and type 1 diabetes mellitus, but not AS.

Ankylosing spondylitis originates from the Greek *ankylos* = bent
+ *spondylos* = vertebra

39. Mitral stenosis

C. Double impulse apex beat

Mitral stenosis occurs as a result of a chronic autoimmune attack upon the mitral valves. This leads to scar tissue formation, which ultimately tethers the leaflets and prevents them from opening fully. The autoimmune attack is usually triggered by rheumatic fever (group A streptococcus) antibodies cross-reacting with endocardial tissue. Mitral stenosis leads to reduced cardiac output and hence peripheral cyanosis. The apex beat is described as "tapping" because of the increased force in closing the mitral valve. The opening snap in diastole correlates to forced opening of the valve and may be followed by a mid-diastolic murmur. Mitral stenosis leads to left atrial enlargement, and this is related to a bifid P-wave (P mitrale) on the ECG. The P-wave is bifid due to the presence of a larger P-wave (left atrium) superimposed on a smaller one (right atrium). Hypertrophic obstructive cardiomyopathy leads to a double impulse apex beat.

40. Management of facial weakness

E. Steroids, antiviral therapy and eye protection

This man appears to have Bell palsy – an *idiopathic* seventh nerve palsy. The fact that the forehead is not spared means that there is lower motor neuron weakness, and the lack of any other neurological symptoms, conditions such as diabetes and vasculitis, or identifiable structural lesion along the path of the seventh nerve, means that the cause is most likely to be idiopathic. It is thought to be an inflammatory process in most cases, causing compression at the facial canal or stylomastoid foramen. Steroids are commonly used in therapy, although the evidence for its efficacy is debated. The same may be said for antiviral therapy. Penicillin-based antibiotics are used in Lyme disease, which is a rare cause of seventh nerve palsy, but there is no evidence of it here (i.e. preceding rash, arthralgia or flu-like symptoms). A dangerous complication of Bell palsy is corneal abrasions, which can happen especially during sleep, and therefore eye protection is recommended. There is no evidence that this man's symptoms were due to an ischaemic event – the onset over a few days, lack of risk factors and lack of other neurology make this evident – and thus aspirin, dipyridamole, statin therapy and an angiotensin-converting enzyme (ACE) inhibitor would all be inappropriate.

Charles Bell, Scottish anatomist (1774-1842)

41. Pathological fracture

C. Multiple myeloma

In multiple myeloma there is malignant proliferation of plasma cells that secrete monoclonal antibodies and light immunoglobulin chains. Multiple myeloma is a multi-system disease that may present with lethargy, bone pain, pathological fracture, renal failure, amyloidosis and pancytopenia due to marrow infiltration. Diagnosis requires two of the following three criteria: 1) marrow plasmacytosis, 2) serum/urinary immunoglobulin-light chains (Bence Jones protein) and 3) skeletal lesions (osteolytic lesions, pepperpot skull and pathological fractures). People who have evidence of serum or urine monoclonal antibodies but do not fulfil the criteria for multiple myeloma are said to have "monoclonal gammopathy of uncertain significance", which has a 2% annual risk of transforming into multiple myeloma. The treatment of multiple myeloma aims to improve symptoms and suppress disease activity. Bone pain may be controlled with analgesia, bisphosphonates and orthopaedic intervention. Renal failure, caused by the deposition of light chains within the kidney, is usually managed by promoting fluid intake although renal replacement therapy may be required. Infection, anaemia and bleeding caused by pancytopenia secondary to marrow infiltration can be managed with broad-spectrum antimicrobials, erythropoietin therapy and blood product replacement, respectively.

In patients younger than 55 years of age, allogeneic stem cell transplantation offers a hope of cure but has a treatment-related mortality rate of 30% and is associated with significant morbidity from treatment-related side effects. Chemotherapy (e.g. mephalan and prednisolone) is often used to suppress disease activity but is generally viewed as palliative. Survival is usually less than 4 years, with death occurring secondary to renal failure or infection.

Henry Bence Jones, English physician (1813-1873)

42. Management of HIV

D. CD4 count <200 cells/mm³

At a CD4 count of <200 cells/mm³, the development of acquired immune deficiency syndrome (AIDS)-related opportunistic infections becomes highly likely (for instance, *Pneumocystis* pneumonia). Therefore it is recommended that below this level, HAART should be started, typically involving two nucleoside analogue reverse transcriptase inhibitors (NRTIs), such as zidovudine and didanosine, and one of either a protease inhibitor such as indinavir or a non-nucleoside reverse transcriptase inhibitor (NNRTI) such as efavirenz. A higher viral load indicates that the CD4 count is likely to fall more rapidly, and a high viral load with a moderately low CD4 count (such as 300 cells/mm³) can be an indicator to start treatment. Viral load alone however does not as accurately predict onset of opportunistic infection and thus guide treatment. Symptoms of an opportunistic infection alone can indicate starting HAART, however, fever and weight loss are non-specific symptoms. The patient should, of course, be investigated for a cause.

43. Tetralogy of Fallot

C. His pulse exhibits a radio-femoral delay

Radio-femoral delay is a symptom of coarctation of the aorta, when the coarctation (narrowing) occurs between the left subclavian artery and the aortic bifurcation. A stenosis higher up between the right brachiocephalic artery and the left subclavian artery can cause asymmetric radial pulses (still with right radio-femoral delay).

Tetralogy of Fallot has four defining malformations:

1. Ventricular septal defect (VSD)
2. Pulmonary stenosis that turns the VSD into a right–left shunt, causing cyanosis; acute attacks (due to increases in pulmonary vascular resistance) can be managed by squatting, which raises peripheral vascular resistance and therefore reduces the right–left shunt
3. Right ventricular hypertrophy
4. Overriding aorta, i.e. the aorta is connected to both ventricles and in this sense acts like a second VSD, above which it sits

Etienne-Louis Arthur Fallot, French physician (1850-1911)

44. Investigation of dysphagia

D. Endoscopy

This pattern of symptoms most closely represents achalasia, which is a dysmotility disorder of the distal oesophagus. In achalasia there is difficulty in swallowing both liquids and solids. A barium swallow is often diagnostic and will show a narrowed distal oesophagus with dilatation of the segment proximal to this (a bird's beak appearance) and a lack of peristalis in this area. Dysphagia lasting more than 3 weeks, however, always warrants an endoscopy to exclude a malignant stricture.

45. Thalassaemia trait

E. No treatment required

This man has only one thalassaemia gene, and is therefore a carrier of the trait. Investigations will show a microcytic hypochromic anaemia with normal ferritin and serum iron, and there will be an increase in A2 haemoglobin on electrophoresis. It is important in order to differentiate this from iron-deficiency anaemia, which may require further investigation in a man of his age. The importance of diagnosis of the thalassaemia trait is to allow genetic counselling.

46. Warfarin therapy

B. Erythromycin

Warfarin is a common anticoagulant that works by inhibiting an essential step in the synthesis of vitamin K-dependent clotting factors (II, VII, IX and X). Anticoagulation is measured using the prothrombin time (PT), which is converted into the INR using the following formula:

$$INR = (measured\ PT/normal\ PT) \wedge ISI$$

...where the international sensitivity index (ISI) is a constant number that represents how the particular manufactured batch of tissue factor used in the lab compares to an internationally standardised sample. It is usual for patients on warfarin to have a target INR of 2–4.5 depending on the condition being treated. Warfarin therapy is complicated and some patients develop an inappropriately high INR, which places them at increased risk of bleeding. The most common causes for developing an inappropriately high INR are dosing errors, accidental overdose and drug interaction. Degradation of warfarin is via cytochrome p450 in the liver, which is a common pathway for many other drugs and is also susceptible to inhibition and enhancement. Drugs that are known to potentiate the action of warfarin include antibiotics (including erythromycin), thyroxine, alcohol, antidepressants, aspirin, amioderone and quinine. In this case it is likely that the antibiotics prescribed for the chest infection increased the action of warfarin, causing a significant rise in INR, which placed the patient at risk of a major bleed from minor trauma. The treatment of an inappropriately high INR depends on the specific circumstances. A moderately high INR with no bleeding can usually be corrected by omitting a dose of warfarin. In situations when the INR is significantly raised without bleeding the warfarin should be omitted and an oral dose of vitamin K prescribed. A high INR associated with active bleeding warrants a dose of oral or intravenous vitamin K plus the administration of a prothrombin complex concentrate such as Beriplex®, which contains the deficient factors II, VII, IX and X. When a prothrombin complex concentrate is not available, fresh–frozen plasma may be used as an alternative.

> Warfarin, named after the Wisconsin Alumni Research Foundation, where it was discovered (Warf) + *arin* (indicating its link with coumarin, the natural compound used to make dicoumarol, another anticoagulant)

47. The painful joint

E. Aspirate the joint fully, send the fluid for urgent Gram stain and culture, take blood cultures, and start empirical intravenous antibiotics immediately

This clinical presentation, with acute monoarthritis and systemic signs suggestive of infection (tachycardia, fever) is septic arthritis until proven otherwise. Empirical intravenous antibiotics should be started as soon as possible, in this instance once joint fluid and blood have been sent for Gram stain and cultures. *Staphylococcus aureus* is the most common cause, and so antibiotics with good Gram-positive cover such as flucloxacillin and fusidic acid are amongst those commonly used, but local guidelines should be consulted or the case should be discussed with a microbiologist. If positive, once sensitivities are back you should change the antibiotics as soon as possible, if required. It is imperative that antibiotics are started as soon as possible as septic arthritis can lead to rapid joint destruction, osteomyelitis and even overwhelming sepsis and death. A source for the infection should be sought and answers to the following questions sought:

1. Has the patient had another infection preceding this?
2. Was there any recent surgery or trauma to the affected joint?
3. Is endocarditis a possibility?
4. Could the patient be immunosuppressed?

Differentials of acute monoarthritis include gout (commonly affecting the first metatarsophalangeal joint), pseudogout and sero-negative inflammatory arthritis.

48. The unresponsive patient (1)

E. Naloxone

This man appears to be haemodynamically stable and there is no concern that that is about to change, so the fluid challenge may be unnecessary. Running some maintenance fluids for now may be indicated as it is not known how long he may be in a coma. A blood sugar reading of 6 is normal so there is no need for the glucose. His temperature is normal, and whilst it is easy to become cold in the resuscitation room, a Bair hugger is not indicated. Flumazenil is an antidote for benzodiazepines, however it is only used if a witnessed overadministration of benzodiazepines occurs or if respiratory depression happens secondary to benzodiazepines – reversal of benzodiazepine action can precipitate seizures or ventricular arrhythmias, and in those patients with a history of seizures, flumazenil must never be used. With this patient, it seems likely that he has taken an opioid overdose – he has pinpoint pupils and a reduced respiratory rate. Boluses of naloxone 0.8–2 mg intravenously every 2 minutes, titrating to patient response and aiming for a GCS of 13–14, would be indicated and could induce a rapid reversal of coma.

49. Vomiting

C. Physiological posseting

Physiological posseting, or the effortless regurgitation of food, is a normal phenomenon in most newborn children. It is especially common in premature babies. Five percent of children will still be doing this at 12 months of age. The reassuring features in this case to rule out the other diagnoses is that he is maintaining his growth projectory and is well in himself. Failure to thrive or being unwell in himself would be the biggest indicator that this is not normal physiological regurgitation.

50. Weight loss

A. Anorexia nervosa

Weight loss in a young girl can herald the start of a malabsorption syndrome or hormonal disturbance such as hyperthyroidism. Every case needs to be treated carefully and a thorough history should point towards either organic or psychological illness. Anorexia nervosa is a very common condition that can often cause overinvestigation in the first instance to reassure the physician. A careful psychological and food history is necessary for diagnosis. Treatment depends on the severity of the illness. Hospitalisation may be required in severe cases. An ECG should be performed to look for any heart strain and a bone scan may be indicated if anorexia lasts for longer than 1 year, to rule out osteoporosis.

Practice Paper 2: Questions

1. Acute confusion

Which of the following routine blood tests is most likely to indicate a cause of an elderly patient's acute confusional state?

A Calcium
B C-reactive protein (CRP)
C Liver function tests
D Sodium
E Urea

2. HLA-B27

Which of the following conditions is not associated with HLA-B27?

A Crohn's disease
B Psoriasis
C Scleritis
D Ulcerative colitis
E Uveitis

3. Heart failure (1)

A 69-year-old man presents with a range of signs and symptoms that give the impression of heart failure.

Which of the following is not a feature of heart failure?

A Hepatomegaly
B Non-pitting oedema
C Pulsus alternans
D Raised jugular venous pressure
E Tricuspid regurgitation

4. Scoring systems (1)

A 57-year-old man with a history of alcohol abuse presents with a 12-hour history of severe central epigastric pain radiating through to the back. Blood tests reveal a normal white cell count, amylase 2250 U/ml, LDH 530 IU/L, calcium 2.2 mmol/L, albumin 38 g/dl, urea 12 mmol/L and blood glucose 14 mmol/L. An arterial blood gas reading demonstrates a pO_2 of 10.2 kPa on room air.

What is his Glasgow score?

A 0
B 1
C 2
D 3
E 4

5. Investigation of headache (1)

A 60-year-old man presents with total visual loss in his left eye that developed over 1 day. He says he had a headache on the left side in the 5 days that preceded the visual loss, which was constant and severe, and worse on talking or eating. On further questioning he said he has been feeling lethargic for the last 2 months and has been having some shoulder aches. There is no relevant past medical history and he has never smoked. On examination, there is no vision in the left eye, there is a relative afferent papillary defect, and the optic disc appears red and swollen on ophthalmoscopy. There is no other cranial nerve defect or neurological defect.

Which investigation would confirm the most likely diagnosis?

A Computed tomography (CT)
B Inflammatory markers (C-reactive protein (CRP), erythrocyte sedimentation rate (ESR))
C Lumbar puncture
D Temporal artery biopsy
E Visual evoked potentials

6. Management of hypercalcaemia

A 70-year-old man presents to the emergency department with a cough productive of blood-stained green sputum and shortness of breath. A chest X-ray demonstrates a suspicious lesion in the right lower zone associated with consolidation. On further questioning, he admits to recent weight loss and back pain. Blood tests show:

Na^+	137 mmol/L	Corrected Ca^{2+}	3.0 mmol/L
K^+	3.8 mmol/L	PO_4	0.33 mmol/L
Urea	14.5 mmol/L	Alk Phos	450 mmol/L
Creatinine	160 µmol/L		

Which of the following is NOT appropriate in the management of this patient?

A Check patient's urea and electrolyte level and serum calcium level twice daily
B Consider starting intravenous bisphosphonate
C Consider starting loop diuretics
D Rehydration with intravenous normal saline
E Request an urgent isotope bone scan

7. Shortness of breath (2)

A 45-year-old woman with type 1 diabetes and rheumatoid arthritis has been admitted after a massive overdose of ibuprofen and has been noted to have acute renal failure with a creatinine level of around 350 μmol/L. The next day, you are called to see her as she is becoming breathless. Her airway is clear. She looks anxious. Her respiratory rate is 28/min and her saturations are 86% on air. You hear bibasal crepitations in her chest, which is slightly dull to percussion at both bases. She has a pulse of 110 bpm and blood pressure of 125/80 mmHg. Her urine output has been 120 ml in the last 10 hours, and you note that her jugular venous pressure is high. It appears from the notes that the night house officer was asked to see her due to her low urine output and prescribed aggressive fluid resuscitation.

What is the most likely reason for her breathlessness?

A Acute respiratory distress syndrome
B Aspiration
C Pleural effusion
D Pneumonia
E Pulmonary oedema

8. Nosebleeds

A 55-year-old man is referred to haematology with repeated nosebleeds, malaise, weight loss and night sweats. Investigations show a raised white cell count, mainly neutrophils and myelocytes, anaemia, increased urate and increased alkaline phosphatase. On blood film there are no blast cells. Genetic studies show a t(9:22) translocation encoding for the *BCR-ABL* gene.

What is his diagnosis?

A Acute lymphoblastic leukaemia
B Acute myeloid leukaemia
C Chronic lymphoblastic leukaemia
D Chronic myeloid leukaemia
E Non-Hodgkin lymphoma

9. Haematemesis

A 48-year-old man is admitted to the emergency department vomiting blood. He has a blood pressure of 80/45 mmHg with a heart rate of 135 bpm. He is cool and clammy to the touch.

Which of the following should NOT be in your immediate management of this patient?

A Alert the endoscopy suite
B Contact senior support
C Cross match 6–8 U blood urgently

D Insert two large-bore cannulae

E Transfer to the ward

10. Failure to thrive

A 5-month-old girl presents with failure to thrive, pallor and mild jaundice. The child has frontal bossing of the skull, prominent maxillae and hepatosplenomegaly.

Which of the following is the most likely diagnosis?

A Congenital biliary atresia

B Congenital hypothyroid

C Hydrops fetalis

D Lead poisoning

E Thalassaemia major

11. Osteoarthritis of the hand

Which of the following findings on hand examination are suggestive of osteoarthritis?

A Dactylitis

B Osteophytes at the distal and/or proximal interphalangeal joints

C Prominent nail fold capillary loops

D Prominent ulnar styloid

E Trigger finger

12. Study design

Several trials have been published regarding the role of therapeutic statin use in bowel cancer. The published results are disparate and you wish to find the best answer from the available literature.

Which of the following study designs would you use?

A Case series

B Delphi method

C Meta-analysis

D Non-systematic review

E Randomised, controlled trial

13. Acute coronary syndrome (2)

A 52-year-old man presents to his GP with chest pain and is afraid he is having a heart attack. His most significant symptom toward a diagnosis of acute coronary syndrome (ACS) is:

A Chest pain located just under the left nipple, near the apex beat

B A past medical history of controlled angina

C A sharp chest pain

D Shortness of breath

E Tachycardia

14. Mouth ulcers

A 29-year-old woman is concerned about recurrent ulcers she gets in her mouth. Occurring every few months, they are small, grey, shallow ulcers that disappear spontaneously. She has no other gastrointestinal symptoms or weight loss.

What is the most likely cause?

A Behçet disease
B Crohn's disease
C Herpes simplex
D Idiopathic aphthous ulcers
E Oral carcinoma

15. Antibiotics (1)

From the following list of antibiotics and their predominant cover, which is incorrect?

A Co-amoxiclav – broad-spectrum Gram-positive and -negative cover
B Flucloxacillin – Gram-positive cover
C Gentamicin – Gram-negative cover
D Metronidazole – anaerobic cover
E Vancomycin – Gram-negative cover

16. Pleural effusion

A 62-year-old Asian woman presents to the emergency department with increasing shortness of breath for the past 2 weeks. She has a past medical history of breast cancer, ischaemic heart disease, previous myocardial infarction with a stent in her left anterior descending artery, and osteoarthritis. On examination, there are reduced breath sounds on her lung bases, and dullness to percussion. Both legs are swollen. A chest X-ray demonstrates a right-sided pleural effusion. A simple aspiration of the pleural cavity showed a pleural fluid protein:serum protein ratio <0.5.

What is the most likely underlying diagnosis?

A Congestive cardiac failure
B Metastatic lung cancer
C Rheumatoid disease
D Systemic lupus erythematosus
E Tuberculosis

17. Topical steroids

A 25-year-old man presents with a severe outbreak of a dry erythematous itchy rash that is now widespread, despite having used a steroid cream prescribed by his GP. It appears to be eczema, and along with regular emollients for the dryness, and antihistamines for the itch, you would like to prescribe some very potent topical steroids for a brief period to attempt get on top of the outbreak.

Which of the following is classed as a very potent topical steroid?

A Betnovate
B Dermovate
C Eumovate
D Hydrocortisone
E Prednisolone

18. Skin lesion (2)

A 7-year-old boy presents with multiple erythematous patches, over both sides of his face, head, neck, upper chest and left arm and shoulder, which appear to be covered in a honey-coloured crust. His mother says that the lesions have spread, over about a week, starting at the left neck and radiating outwards. The child appears to be upset and the lesions are itchy. There is no past medical history and no history of recent infections.

Which of the following diagnoses is most likely?

A Eczema
B Erysipelas
C Impetigo
D Psoriasis
E Staphylococcal scalded skin syndrome

19. Management of Parkinson's disease (2)

A 75-year-old man has been recently diagnosed with Parkinson's disease and started on levodopa (L-DOPA), which has helped his tremor and bradykinesia significantly. However, in the past week he had a fall shortly after getting out of his chair, during which he briefly blacked out, and afterwards was sweating and felt cold.

Which of the following side effects most likely explains the fall?

A Dyskinesia
B Hallucinations
C Nausea
D None, he actually has multiple system atrophy and not Parkinson's disease
E Postural hypotension

20. Arrhythmias

You are reviewing the medication of a 62-year-old man suffering from depression and cardiac arrhythmias. He was recently discharged from hospital for chest pain. During his admission, he was noted to have "torsades de pointes".

What is torsades de pointes?

A A clinical sign associated with acute pericarditis
B A congenital facial sign associated with congenital heart defects
C A form of ventricular tachycardia that can self-correct but can also lead to sudden death
D A variation in the QRS that changes in magnitude with inspiration and expiration
E Alternate T-wave inversion

21. Back pain

A 69-year-old man recently diagnosed with metastatic prostate cancer presents with weakness in his legs and urinary retention. He has had back pain for years but in the last 24 hours this has become very severe in his lower back. On examination he has a sensory deficit, loss of anal tone and poor sensation in the skin around the anus. When catheterised he has a residual volume of 1.5 L.

Which of the following is the most informative initial investigation?

A Computed tomography (CT) of the abdomen/pelvis
B Lumbar X-rays
C Magnetic resonance imaging (MRI) of the lumbar spine
D Serum calcium
E Ultrasound scan (USS) of the renal tract

22. Bruising in children

A 6-year-old boy has a 1-month history of aching bones and muscle pains. On examination he appears pale and has multiple bruises along his legs. He has extensive lymphadenopathy. Blast cells are seen on the blood film.

What is the most likely diagnosis?

A Acute lymphoblastic leukaemia
B Child abuse
C Henoch–Schönlein purpura
D Juvenile idiopathic arthritis
E Sickle cell disease

23. Management of skin lesions (2)

A 76-year-old man presents with a vesicular eruption on the left side of his forehead only. It is severely painful and the vesicles have started to crust over. On examination, the area affected is well-demarcated. You also note a red eye with apparent conjunctivitis.

Given the most likely diagnosis, which of the following treatments is the most appropriate?

A Intravenous aciclovir
B Oral aciclovir
C Topical aciclovir
D Topical antibiotic
E Topical steroids

24. Coarctation of the aorta

You find a loud systolic murmur in a 14-year-old girl during a preoperative assessment for an appendicectomy.

Which of the following signs or investigations do NOT help confirm a diagnosis of coarctation of the aorta?

A Ankle brachial pressure index
B Electrocardiogram
C Magnetic resonance angiography
D Radial pulse asymmetry
E Radio-femoral delay

25. Management of asthma (2)

A 28-year-old woman with a past medical history of asthma has been using her inhaled salbutamol more frequently of late. She is currently on an inhaled short-acting beta-2 agonist and an inhaled steroid 800 µg/day. She has been compliant.

What should you do?

A Add inhaled long-acting beta-2 agonist
B Add leukotriene receptor antagonist
C Add oral steroid
D Increase dose of inhaled steroid
E Prescribe inhaled short-acting beta-2 agonist as regular therapy

26. Collapse (2)

A 62-year-old woman presents to the emergency department with collapse. She felt dizzy when she tried to stand up from a sitting position. She did not lose consciousness. She denied any visual disturbances, headache or head injury. She also complained of fatigue over the past month. She takes only omeprazole and paracetamol. An electrocardiogram (ECG) showed normal sinus rhythm. Her blood pressure was 102/50 mmHg. A blood test revealed the following: Na^+ 126 mmol/L, K^+ 6.5 mmol/L, urea 10.0 mmol/L, and creatinine 139 µmol/L.

What is the most likely diagnosis?

A Acromegaly
B Adrenal insufficiency
C Cushing's disease
D Hypocalcaemia
E Hypothyroidism

27. Diagnosis of abdominal pain (2)

A 56-year-old man with a long history of alcohol abuse presents to the emergency department with abdominal pain. On examination he has a distended abdomen with shifting dullness and has a temperature of 38.2°C.

What is the most likely diagnosis?

A Bowel obstruction
B Liver cirrhosis
C Mallory–Weiss syndrome
D Perforated peptic ulcer
E Spontaneous bacterial peritonitis (SBP)

28. Investigation of stroke

A 52-year-old man with hyperthyroidism, vitiligo and a 30 pack/year smoking history, presents to hospital with an acute clumsiness of his right hand. Neurological examination reveals normal cranial nerves, and the only abnormal feature on the limb examination is some past pointing and dysdiadochokinesis in the right hand. Diffusion-weighted magnetic resonance imaging (MRI) reveals a small right-sided cerebellar infarct.

Which of the following investigations is unlikely to be helpful?

A Carotid Doppler
B Electrocardiogram (ECG)
C Erythrocyte sedimentation rate (ESR)
D Full blood count
E Magnetic resonance angiography

29. Diagnosis of cough (2)

A 32-year-old woman presents to the GP with a 3-month history of non-productive cough and breathlessness on exertion. She also complains of fatigue, weight loss and joint pain. She smokes 15 cigarettes/day. She has not travelled to any foreign countries recently. On examination, fine interstitial crackles are heard on the anterior chest wall. There are multiple tender red lumps on both shins.

What is the most likely diagnosis?

A Idiopathic pulmonary fibrosis
B Lung cancer
C Sarcoidosis
D Systemic lupus erythematosus
E Wegener granulomatosis

30. Diagnosis of multiple sclerosis (2)

Which of the following findings on lumbar puncture is most commonly used to suggest a diagnosis of multiple sclerosis (given a correlative clinical picture)?

A Autoantibodies to myelin basic protein
B Oligoclonal bands on electrophoresis
C Presence of red blood cells
D Raised lymphocytes
E Raised protein

31. Investigation of abdominal pain

A 59-year-old woman with known polycythaemia vera presents to the emergency department with right upper quadrant pain, tender hepatomegaly and gross ascites, which has come on suddenly. There is no jaundice.

What is the next most appropriate investigation?

A Cytomegalovirus (CMV) screen
B Gamma-glutamyl transferase (GGT) levels
C Hepatitis serology
D Hepatic vein Doppler ultrasound scan (USS)
E Human immunodeficiency virus (HIV) testing

32. Diagnosis of cough (3)

A 60-year-old Chinese man presents to the GP with a 4-month history of weight loss. He has lost around 1 stone in weight. He also has a cough productive of green sputum without blood. He has a reduced appetite, insomnia and night sweats. His past medical history includes hypertension and ischaemic heart disease. He is a retired managing director who has just emigrated from Hong Kong to England. He denies a smoking history. His observations include temperature 36.4°C, pulse 67 bpm, blood pressure 152/92 mmHg and respiratory rate 15/min. On examination, there is dullness to percussion over the left upper lung zone.

What is the most likely diagnosis?

A Lung cancer
B Lung abscess
C Pulmonary infarction
D Tuberculosis
E Wegener granulomatosis

33. Diagnosis of tuberculosis

A 27-year-old man presents with a 3-month history of cough with some blood streaking, loss of weight and night sweats. You suspect tuberculosis.

Which of the following chest X-ray findings is not consistent with tuberculosis?

A Cavitating lesion
B Consolidation of a lobe
C Diffuse 1–2 mm spots of increased opacity
D Perihilar ground-glass changes
E Pleural effusion

34. Thrombocytopenia

A 74-year-old man is admitted to hospital with an acute-on-chronically ischaemic leg and started on intravenous heparin. Blood tests taken 5 days later show platelet levels have dropped from 250 to 54×10^9.

What is the most likely cause for thrombocytopenia in this patient?

A Chronic lymphocytic leukaemia
B Disseminated intravascular coagulation
C Evans syndrome
D Heparin-induced thrombocytopenia (HIT)
E Thrombotic thrombocytopenic purpura

35. Meningitis

A 40-year-old man presents to the emergency department after 8 hours of a severe frontal headache, photophobia and two episodes of vomiting. On examination his Glasgow Coma Score (GCS) is 13 (eyes open to voice, verbal response with confused sentences, and moving freely), he has a temperature of 38.5°C, a BP of 95/65 mmHg and pulse rate of 105 bpm. He is photophobic and has neck stiffness. There is no rash and no focal neurological deficit as far as you can ascertain. His wife is present and is able to elaborate on the history. He has hit the bottle quite hard since losing his job 7 months ago and has been drinking 8–10 cans of lager per night. He has recently been coughing a lot and feeling unwell. He still lives at home and has not appeared to lose weight recently.

What are you most concerned that this might be?

A *Listeria* meningitis
B Meningococcal meningitis
C Pneumococcal meningitis
D Tubercular meningitis
E Viral meningitis

36. Electrocardiogram (2)

A 63-year-old male smoker, on diuretics for essential hypertension, presents to the emergency department with chest pain. His ECG is presented to you. Amongst other signs, you notice T-wave inversion.

Which of the following does not cause T-wave inversion?

A Hyperkalaemia
B Left bundle branch block
C Left ventricular hypertrophy
D Myocardial infarction
E Myocardial ischaemia

37. Diarrhoea (2)

A 72-year-old man is bed-bound following a severe stroke several years previously and lives in a nursing home with full-time care. The staff noticed that over the last 8 days he didn't pass any stool motions until this morning, when there was profuse, offensive liquid stool. They are concerned this may be infective diarrhoea. On examination there is hard stool in the rectum.

What is the most likely diagnosis?

A *Campylobacter* infection
B Carcinoma of the rectum
C Inflammatory bowel disease
D Norovirus
E Overflow diarrhoea

38. Management of epilepsy

A 24-year-old man presents with two episodes of involuntary clonic beating of the right arm followed by loss of consciousness with urinary and faecal incontinence. He then had a headache and confusion for some hours (no-one witnessed any episode). A diagnosis of motor partial seizures with secondary generalisation is made. He is started on valproate.

Which of the following would you NOT tell him (as it is untrue)?

A Computed tomography (CT)/magnetic resonance imaging (MRI) is indicated to look for a cause
B No driving for 1 year after the last seizure
C On valproate, blood tests will need to be monitored for liver enzymes and full blood count
D Valproate may cause gum hypertrophy
E Valproate may cause hair loss

39. Diagnosis of HIV-related illness

A 42-year-old woman with known HIV presents with a 3-week history of dry cough and increasing breathlessness. She is now unable to walk 100 yards without becoming short of breath. You suspect pneumocystis pneumonia.

Which of the following tests is the best way to confirm the diagnosis?

A Bronchoalveolar lavage
B Chest X-ray
C Computed tomography (CT) of the chest
D Cytology of sputum induced by nebulised hypertonic saline
E Hypoxaemia on arterial blood gas

40. Tiredness

A 65-year-old woman presents to her GP complaining of tiredness, shortness of breath and loss of sensation in her feet. On examination she is visibly pale, has mild jaundice and glossitis. She has loss of joint position sense and vibration distally, with extensor plantar reflexes, absent ankle jerks and brisk knee jerks bilaterally.

What is the most likely cause for her symptoms?

A Chronic sickle cell disease
B G6PD deficiency
C Heart failure
D Renal failure
E Vitamin B_{12} deficiency

41. Management of acne (1)

A 17-year-old girl shuffles awkwardly into clinic with her mother, who explains that her daughter has suffered from severe acne for the last few years and nothing that the GP has tried has shifted it. On examination, as well as several large pustules on her face and comedones, some scarring is beginning to develop. You would like to start oral isotretinoin (roaccutane).

When counselling about side effects, which of the following would you NOT advise the patient?

A Blood tests should be taken to monitor for hyperlipidaemia
B Blood tests should be taken to monitor for raised liver function tests
C Most people feel depressed on isotretinoin
D Parts of the skin and lips often get very dry
E Pregnancy should be avoided as teratogenicity is a risk

42. Epigastric pain (2)

A 68-year-old man presents with a 3-month history of epigastric pain and weight loss. He has a history of acid reflux, which his GP has been managing.

What is the next most appropriate step?

A Computed tomography (CT) scan of the abdomen
B Dietician review
C Increase his proton pump inhibitor (PPI) and ask him to return in 1 month if symptoms don't settle
D Treat empirically for *H. pylori* infection and review in 1 month
E Upper gastrointestinal (GI) endoscopy

43. Sexually transmitted infections (1)

A 23-year-old man develops a urethral discharge and dysuria after a recent change of sexual partner and urethral swabs are positive for *Chlamydia*.

Which of the following statements about antibiotic treatment is TRUE?

A His partners should be asked about symptoms and tested only if symptomatic
B His partners should be tested for *Chlamydia* and treated only if positive
C His partners should be tested for *Chlamydia* and treated with antibiotics regardless of outcome
D No antibiotic treatment is necessary provided he abstains from having sexual intercourse for 2 weeks
E Only the patient who has presented needs antibiotic therapy

44. Non-steroidal anti-inflammatories

A 75-year-old woman is suffering from osteoarthritis of the hips and knees and paracetamol is not touching the pain. You want to consider use of a non-steroidal anti-inflammatory drug (NSAID).

Which of the following is NOT a relative or absolute contraindication to NSAID use?

A Asthma
B Concomitant aspirin use
C Concomitant steroid use
D Congestive cardiac failure
E Previous gastric ulcers

45. Renal transplantation

Which of the following is NOT a contraindication to renal transplantation?

A Active tuberculosis
B High-pressure urinary tract, e.g. posterior urethral valves
C Malignancy
D Severe arterial disease with stenosed iliac vessels
E Severe ischaemic heart disease with unstable angina and congestive cardiac failure

46. Thrombolysis in ischaemic stroke

Which of the following patients is eligible for thrombolysis with intravenous recombinant tissue plasminogen activator?

A 2 hours post onset, BP 150/80 mmHg, GCS 11, MRI shows infarct
B 2 hours post onset, BP 160/90 mmHg, GCS 15, MRI shows haemorrhage
C 2 hours post onset, BP 160/95 mmHg, GCS 15, MRI shows infarct
D 2 hours post onset, BP 195/115 mmHg, GCS 15, MRI shows infarct
E 7 hours post onset, BP 135/80 mmHg, GCS 15, MRI shows infarct

47. Diagnosis of chest pain (2)

A 43-year-old woman presents with an acute sharp, central chest pain radiating to the left arm that is worse on inspiration and at night. She reports that it is preventing her coughing which, in turn, is prolonging a recent chest infection. On examination, her chest exhibits vesicular breath sounds with bi-basal crackles. Her electrocardiogram (ECG) shows widespread concave ST elevation in sinus rhythm.

Which of the following is the most likely diagnosis?

A Acute pericarditis
B Cardiac tamponade

C Pulmonary embolism
D ST-elevated myocardial infarction
E Unstable angina

48. Management of oliguria (2)

An 87-year-old man with a background of Alzheimer's disease, a previous stroke, and atrial fibrillation (for which he is on warfarin), is admitted with increasing amounts of painless haematuria. He is catheterised and the warfarin stopped. The haematuria reduces and then seems to stop. Problems with his residential home are delaying discharge. You note 2 days later that his creatinine level has risen to 250 µmol/L. When you go to see him, he seems stable, as do his observations. He does seem slightly dry with reduced skin turgor and delayed capillary refill. The urine output has not been carefully documented in the last few days, and by your calculations, 100 ml have been passed in the last 24 hours. On examination he appears to have a mass in his central lower abdomen.

What should be your next step?

A Fluid challenge of 500 ml normal saline over 10 minutes
B Flush the catheter with 50 ml warm saline and then aspirate
C Insert a suprapubic catheter
D Remove the catheter
E Request an ultrasound of the urinary tract

49. The unresponsive patient (2)

A 70-year-old woman presents with hip pain following a fall. The fall appears to have been related to alcohol ingestion and, whilst the history is vague, she denies loss of consciousness and does not seem grossly confused, nor is there evidence of infection. She is a smoker and has a history of ischaemic heart disease and depression. A hip fracture is ruled out and she is admitted for rehabilitation purposes. On day 3, however, the nurses report that she is increasingly sleepy and muddled. On examination, observations are stable, she is apyrexial, her Glasgow Coma Score (GCS) is 12, and on neurological examination, she appears to have some mild left arm and leg weakness with normal or brisk reflexes. There is no hemianopia or other neurological deficit.

Which of the following is most likely to explain the changes?

A Bacterial meningitis
B Intracerebral haemorrhage
C Lacunar infarct
D Subarachnoid haemorrhage
E Subdural haematoma

50. Thyrotoxicosis

A 40-year-old woman presents to the GP with a history of weight loss and irritability. She has lost 1 stone in the past 2 weeks. She claims that she has a normal appetite. She also complains of blurring of the vision for the past month. On examination, she has a "staring look" with lid lag and lid retraction.

What is the most likely diagnosis?

A Graves' disease
B Hashimoto thyroiditis
C Multinodular goitre
D Myasthenia gravis
E Toxic thyroid adenoma

Practice Paper 2: Answers

1. Acute confusion

B. C-reactive protein (CRP)

The most common cause of acute confusional state in elderly patients is a chest or urinary tract infection. These may present atypically, without overt symptoms or a temperature, so looking for a rise in CRP roughly corresponding with the onset of confusion can suggest that performing a septic screen (blood cultures, chest X-ray, urine dipstick and culture) would be of use in finding the cause. Uraemia, liver failure, hyponatraemia, and hyper- or hypocalcaemia can cause acute confusional state, but more rarely than an infection in older patients.

2. HLA-B27

C. Scleritis

Inflammatory bowel disease is associated with HLA-B27, as is psoriasis. Uveitis is inflammation of the iris and associated structures, and causes acute pain with blurred vision and photophobia with reddening of the iris. This is associated with both ankylosing spondylitis and HLA-B27. Scleritis is inflammation of the sclera, causing pain and a gritty sensation in the eye with redness of the sclera. This is associated with connective tissue disorders and rheumatoid arthritis. If left untreated this can cause perforation of the eye. It is not associated with HLA-B27. Genetic testing for HLA-B27 can be useful in difficult diagnostic cases for seronegative spondyloarthropathies and in counselling patients regarding chances of their offspring developing the same disease.

3. Heart failure (1)

B. Non-pitting oedema

Heart failure is a disease of chronic, insidious onset that can first present with shortness of breath, persistent cough or insomnia. The heart fails to maintain adequate cardiac output for a variety of reasons; the harder it tries, the faster it fails. Occasionally, the left ventricle will weaken to the point where it cannot empty efficiently. The subsequent raised end-diastolic volume causes a pre-stretched ventricle, leading to a more forceful contraction (Starling's law). This alternating strong–weak pattern can be seen in the ECG as pulsus alternans (varying amplitudes of the R-wave). A column of blood builds up proximal to the left ventricle, in the lungs, causing pulmonary oedema. This creates afterload upon the right ventricle, which can lead to tricuspid regurgitation. The bottleneck of blood can extend further, through the right side of the heart and hence JVP is raised (the heart is unable to pull all the blood from the jugular vein through the lungs and the left ventricle). Furthermore, close to the right side of the heart, the inferior vena cava remains full of blood, leading to oedema in the liver (hepatomegaly). Ankle veins swell with blood as the heart fails to suck the blood vertically against gravity. The increased hydrostatic pressure results in fluid extravasation into tissues. The push of a finger is enough to displace this tissue fluid, hence this ankle oedema is pitting. Causes of non-pitting oedema include lymphoedema and pretibial myxoedema.

Oedema, from Greek *oedema* = swelling

4. Scoring systems (1)

C. 2

The massively raised amylase with this clinical picture supports a diagnosis of acute pancreatitis. Acute pancreatitis can be a life-threatening condition for it is an unpredictable disease that can cause quick deterioration. To aid management, the modified Glasgow criteria were devised to help prognosis and triage patients to an appropriate level of care. The eight parts of the Glasgow criteria are as follows (1 point for each):

Age	>55 years
White cell count	$>15 \times 10^3/\mu L$
Urea	>16 mmol/L
Glucose	>10 mmol/L
Arterial pO_2	<8 kPa
Albumin	<32 mmol/L
Calcium	<2.0 mmol/L
Lactate dehydrogenase	>600 mmol/L

This man scores 2 for age and his raised blood sugar, which is a moderate risk for pancreatitis. A score of 3 and above should indicate to the physician the need to discuss the case with intensive care as these patients are more likely to need invasive monitoring of their fluid balance. Patients should ideally be re-scored 48 hours after admission.

5. Investigation of headache (1)

D. Temporal artery biopsy

The most likely diagnosis here is temporal arteritis, or giant cell arteritis. The preceding constant severe headache with jaw claudication is classic. The man may also have polymyalgia rheumatica (PMR), which is estimated to co-exist in 20% of cases. The question asks for the investigation to confirm the diagnosis, which is the biopsy of the temporal artery. Inflammatory markers will be raised, adding to the clinical picture, but this is rather general. Visual evoked potentials will tell that the axons of the optic nerve have been damaged, but that won't delineate the cause. Lumbar puncture is unlikely to tell anything specific or helpful, and CT is not useful at looking at soft tissue damage or inflammation.

6. Management of hypercalcaemia

E. Request an urgent isotope bone scan

The most common causes of hypercalcaemia are primary hyperparathyroidism and malignant hypercalcaemia. Patients with hypercalcaemia present with polyuria, polydipsia, renal colic, nausea, anorexia, lethargy, dyspepsia, peptic ulceration, constipation, depression, drowsiness and impaired cognition. Urgent fluid replacement with 0.9% saline is essential (3–6 L over 24 hours) and the patient's urea and electrolyte, and calcium levels should be checked twice daily. Loop diuretics could aid renal clearance of calcium. Intravenous bisphosphonate (e.g. pamidronate) could cause a fall in calcium by causing bone reabsorption. Its effect is maximal at 2–3 days and lasts a few weeks.

7. Shortness of breath (2)

E. Pulmonary oedema

Acute respiratory distress syndrome occurs when inflammatory cytokines and/or lung injury causes capillary permeability to increase and non-fluid overload-related pulmonary oedema. In this case there was no known preceding lung injury and no systemic acute precipitant such as sepsis, shock, haemorrhage or transfusion. The findings of bibasal crackles, however, are consistent with oedema and, whilst the diagnosis is not the most parsimonious, it cannot be entirely ruled out. There has been no vomiting reported to suggest aspiration. A pleural effusion would give stony dull percussion and reduced air entry. This patient is clearly fluid overloaded and so there may be small effusions, but these are unlikely to be the chief cause of breathlessness. The patient is afebrile, and the symmetrical pattern to the crackles goes against (but needn't rule out) a pneumonia. The patient is in acute renal failure, likely secondary to a combination of the long-term use of non-steroidal anti-inflammatory drugs (NSAIDs) (she has rheumatoid arthritis) and the recent NSAID overdose, with a background of diabetes. She is fluid overloaded (note the raised JVP), and the busy overnight house officer probably presumed the low urine output and raised creatinine level was due to dehydration (it appears they didn't read the notes fully) and thus has contributed to the situation. The bibasal crepitations are indicative of pulmonary oedema.

The patient should be placed in a sitting position and wear an oxygen mask, given an opiate such as morphine or diamorphine (to relieve anxiety and also to act as a vasodilator and pool fluid away from the lungs), and given some intravenous furosemide – 40 mg *stat* is a normal dose to try, however due to the renal impairment more may be needed. Response can be gauged by the urine output. Informing the registrar would be essential. Nitrates can also be used – glyceryl nitrite (GTN) spray can be given before starting a nitrate infusion (if the systolic blood pressure is above 90 mmHg). Nitrates again act as a vasodilator and venodilator and pool blood away from the lungs. Pulmonary oedema is a common complication of acute renal failure. Once therapy is initiated, a portable chest X-ray should be ordered to confirm or deny the diagnosis. Further treatment of non-responders includes continuous positive airway pressure (CPAP), and refractory pulmonary oedema is one of the indications for haemofiltration or dialysis in acute renal failure.

8. Nosebleeds

D. Chronic myeloid leukaemia

The t(9:22) translocation (i.e. a translocation between chromosomes 9 and 22) encoding for the *BCR-ABL* gene is also known as the Philadelphia chromosome and is the genetic mutation in over 90% of the cases of chronic myeloid leukaemia. The mutation is a balanced translocation, which leads to increased tyrosine kinase activity disturbing stem cell kinetics.

Chronic myeloid leukaemia (CML) is a myeloproliferative disorder. Its peak incidence is 50–70 years and it is rare in children. There is excessive proliferation of myeloid cells in the bone marrow. Patients typically have massive splenomegaly, anaemia, bruising and infection on a background of generalised illness. A blood film shows myeloblasts (granulocyte precursors) and granulocytosis. Patients with CML but without the Philadelphia chromosome have a worse prognosis compared to those with the translocation. There are three stages of disease in CML: 1) the chronic phase (which is responsive to treatment), 2) the accelerated phase (where the disease is difficult to control) and 3) the blast crisis phase (where the disease progresses into an acute leukaemia, usually AML). The median survival rate is 5 years. Death usually occurs within months of blast transformation (from bleeding and infection). Chemotherapy is often used and allogeneic stem cell transplantation can provide a cure. Having isolated the gene there is now an effective drug that can block the *BCR-ABL* gene – imatinib mesylate – which can reverse the effects of the protein and produce remission in 95% of patients with this mutation.

9. Haematemesis

E. Transfer to the ward

This case presents a young man who is in hypovolaemic shock following a large upper gastrointestinal (GI) bleed. Immediate management in these cases is vital to improving mortality, which is currently about 10% for major bleeds. The aetiology includes gastric or duodenal ulcers, burst oesophageal varices and Mallory–Weiss tears. Initial management relies on effective resuscitation of the patient. Always start with ABC, securing the airway, giving supplementary oxygen, and two large cannulae to ensure rapid fluid infusion is possible. Blood products are the best resuscitative agents – always try to replace like with like – but while you await a cross-match use a colloid infusion or O-negative blood. A catheter should be inserted early during the resuscitation as urine output is a very sensitive marker of renal perfusion. This patient needs to be in a monitored bed while he remains shocked, and so transfer to a ward would not normally be appropriate. Following resuscitation your next actions will depend on aetiology, but if variceal bleeding is suspected an urgent endoscopy and sclerotherapy or banding will be necessary. Alerting the necessary teams at the time of presentation can save vital minutes and ensure that you have the support you need around you.

10. Failure to thrive

E. Thalassaemia major

Beta-thalassaemia major is an autosomal recessive disorder in which there is a complete lack of production of the haemoglobin chain beta-globin. It occurs mainly in Mediterranean and Middle Eastern families and is due to a point mutation on chromosome 11. Because patients with beta-thalassaemia major have mutations on both alleles and cannot synthesise any beta-globin, they cannot produce functioning adult haemoglobin (HbA – $\alpha_2\beta_2$). This condition typically presents within the first year of life, when the production of fetal haemoglobin (HbF – $\alpha_2\gamma_2$) begins to fall. Affected children become generally unwell and fail to thrive secondary to a severe microcytic anaemia. Ferritin levels are normal since there is no iron deficiency. A compensatory increase in the synthesis of HbF and haemoglobin A2 (HbA2 – $\alpha_2\delta_2$) occurs, which can be detected on serum electrophoresis.

Clinical features include failure to thrive, lethargy, pallor and jaundice. On examination there is often hepatosplenomegaly (secondary to extramedullary haematopoiesis) with bossing of the skull, maxillary prominence and long bone deformity (due to excessive intramedullary haematopoiesis). The treatment of beta-thalassaemia major is with regular blood transfusions, aiming to maintain the haemoglobin concentration above 10 g/dL, or with allogenic bone marrow transplant. Regular iron chelation therapy (with desferrioxamine) is required to prevent iron overload and deposition in vital organs such as the heart, liver and endocrine glands. If untreated, death is inevitable in the first years of life.

Beta-thalassaemia minor describes people heterozygous for the beta-chain chromosomal mutation. Affected persons have only mild anaemia and are usually asymptomatic. Alpha-thalassaemia is common in South-East Asia. There are four alpha genes, and therefore four variants of alpha-thalassaemia. Affected patients can be asymptomatic (one gene corruption), have mild hypochromic anaemia (two corruptions), have HbH disease (three corruptions) or can die *in utero* (all four genes are corrupted). HbH is a beta-chain tetramer that is functionally useless. Treatment options are as for beta-thalassaemia.

> Thalassaemia, from Greek *thalassa* = sea + *haima* = blood. It is so-called as the disease is especially prevalent in countries by the sea (i.e. the Mediterranean)

11. Osteoarthritis of the hand

B. Osteophytes at the distal and/or proximal interphalangeal joints

Dactylitis simply means inflammation of the digit(s). Dactylitis can be seen in psoriatic arthropathy – the red, swollen, tender fingers are sometimes referred to as "sausage fingers". Osteophytes at the distal interphalangeal joints are called Heberden nodes and are characteristic of osteoarthritis. Bouchard nodes are osteophytes at the proximal interphalangeal joints and usually appear later than Heberden nodes. Prominent nail fold capillary loops are one of the many skin manifestations of dermatomyositis, an inflammatory disease of the muscle that also affects the skin and is commonly paraneoplastic (i.e. related to an underlying tumour). The prominent ulnar styloid is a change seen in rheumatoid arthritis, which is caused by radial deviation at the wrist joint. Trigger finger is often seen in psoriatic arthritis and rheumatoid arthritis, and its aetiology is not entirely clear, but involves disparity between the flexor tendon and its sheath, which prevent extension of the finger. The finger can suddenly snap back into extension, hence the label "trigger finger". Corticosteroid injection should be tried and is effective in many cases, failing which surgery can release the tendon from its sheath.

> William Heberden, English physician (1710-1801)
>
> Charles-Joseph Bouchard, French pathologist (1837-1915)

12. Study design

C. Meta-analysis

A meta-analysis combines the results of several studies that have looked at a similar hypothesis. By combining the results of multiple data sets, the statistical power of the outcome is increased and the validity of the conclusion improved.

> The Delphi method involves discussion of a topic amongst a focus group of experts in order to arrive at the most agreed-upon solution. As such, it is a poor form of evidence!
>
> Delphi, from the Oracle of Delphi, an ancient Greek shrine (c. 1400 BC) where people travelled to ask prophesy from Pythia, the priestess of Apollo

13. Acute coronary syndrome (2)

B. A past medical history of controlled angina

ACS typically presents with a central/retro sternal chest pain of a crushing character. Stable angina can evolve into the unstable angina of ACS. Tachycardia and shortness of breath are more likely attributed to anxiety in a patient who is scared. It should be noted that these symptoms should never be ignored. Patients in the midst of real cardiac pain are also likely to be anxious and may not necessarily offer textbook characterisations of what they are experiencing. A brief admission to monitor troponin levels 8–12 hours after symptom onset is the correct course of action for any patient presenting with possible cardiac chest pain.

14. Mouth ulcers

D. Idiopathic aphthous ulcers

Aphthous mouth ulcers are a common idiopathic benign condition affecting up to 20% of the population. The incidence rises dramatically in the presence of inflammatory bowel disease. Although very painful, recurrent aphthous ulcers in the absence of gastrointestinal symptoms in a young person are likely to be benign. In recurrent and severe cases it may be appropriate to do blood investigations including serum B_{12} and folate. In cases of a single prolonged ulcer of greater than 3 weeks' duration it is prudent to take a biopsy to exclude a carcinoma. Treatment is symptomatic with topical analgesic agents.

> Aphthous, from Greek *aphtha* = eruption

15. Antibiotics (1)

E. Vancomycin – Gram-negative cover

Vancomycin is a glycopeptide antibiotic that binds D-ala-D-ala peptide sequences to prevent peptidoglycan cell wall synthesis, therefore it is active against Gram-positive but not Gram-negative bacteria (the peptidoglycan cell wall is a far more prominent and important feature in Gram-positive bacteria). Co-amoxiclav has good Gram-positive and -negative cover as well as much anaerobic cover, so is a widely used antibiotic in many scenarios, however, its broad-spectrum characteristic means it disturbs the gut flora and can predispose to *Clostridium difficile* infection. Flucloxacillin is a narrow-spectrum antibiotic with only Gram-positive cover and is often used in staphylococcal infections. Gentamicin has predominantly Gram-negative cover although it has some Gram-positive cover. Metronidazole has wide anaerobic cover and is often used in surgery due to the presence of anaerobes in the bowel.

Hans Christian Joachim Gram, Danish bacteriologist (1853-1938)

Vancomycin, derived from "vanquish"

16. Pleural effusion

A. Congestive cardiac failure

Pleural effusion is characterised by the accumulation of serous fluid within the pleural space. Pleural effusion is categorised into exudative effusion (increased microvascular pressure due to disease of the pleural surface, or injury in the adjacent lung) and transudative effusion (increased hydrostatic pressure or decreased osmotic pressure). Light's criteria states that pleural fluid is an exudate if one or more of the following criteria are met: 1) pleural fluid protein:serum protein ratio >0.5, 2) pleural fluid LDH:serum LDH ratio >0.6, and 3) pleural fluid LDH >two-thirds of the upper limit of normal serum LDH. The causes of exudative effusions include tuberculosis, pneumonia, malignant diseases, pulmonary infarction, rheumatoid disease, systemic lupus erythematosus and acute pancreatitis. The causes of transudative effusions include heart failure, renal failure, liver failure and hypoalbuminaemia.

17. Topical steroids

B. Dermovate

Topical steroids are categorised as mild, moderate, potent, or very potent. The more potent the steroid, the more likely it is to have side effects such as skin atrophy, striae and increased risk of infection. Subsequently, the more potent the topical steroid, the less time it should be used for. Hydrocortisone is a mild steroid, eumovate a moderate steroid, betnovate a potent steroid, and dermovate is a very potent steroid. Prednisolone is an oral steroid, and if the dermovate does not get on top of the eczema, there may be a case for using systemic oral steroids – although they are not normally used in eczema and carry a greater risk of side effects when used: patients can become cushingoid, hypertensive, diabetic, immunosuppressed, osteoporotic, and may develop steroid-induced psychosis.

18. Skin lesion (2)

C. Impetigo

Itchy erythematous skin could be due to a number of things, including eczema and psoriasis, but two features another diagnosis. Firstly, the spreading from a starting point, rather than patches appearing at the same time or cropping up in unrelated positions over time, suggests infection. Secondly, the honey or golden crust is a purulent discharge. Both features are classical of impetigo. Impetigo is a contagious, superficial infection caused most commonly by *Staphylococcus aureus*. The infection spreads when lesions burst to release an exudate, which spreads the bacteria outwards and leaves behind the crust. Swabs should be taken for microscopy, culture, and most importantly sensitivities. In contained infections, topical antibiotics can be prescribed, but in more widespread disease, systemic antibiotics should be used. Antibiotics with good activity against Staphylococci, such as flucloxacillin, should be used pending sensitivities. Antihistamines can be prescribed to help with itching. Underlying skin disease, such as eczema, can predispose.

Erysipelas is a superficial form of cellulitis with a well-demarcated edge to the patch of warm, tender erythema. It can spread more rapidly. Staphylococcal scalded skin syndrome follows infection with group 2 coagulase-positive staphylococci, and a circulating toxin causes epidermal splitting in the granular layer, leading to peeling of the epidermis in large sections. A focus of infection should be sought, and systemic flucloxacillin should be started. It normally develops over a period of hours to days.

Impetigo, from Latin *impetere* = to assail

19. Management of Parkinson's disease (2)

E. Postural hypotension

The fall happened soon after he stood up, involved a brief loss of consciousness, and he had an excess sympathetic discharge shortly afterwards. It certainly sounds like an episode of postural hypotension. Standing up requires a significant degree of autonomic nervous system function to detect and react to the intravascular volume redistribution. As L-DOPA is a precursor in the synthesis of not only dopamine but also noradrenaline, excess peripheral noradrenaline and dopamine can cause widespread autonomic dysfunction, symptoms of which include nausea and postural hypotension. Hallucinations can occur with L-DOPA but are unlikely to cause a fall, and dyskinetic movements could cause a fall but don't explain the loss of consciousness. Multiple system atrophy (MSA), a Parkinson-plus syndrome, indeed includes prominent autonomic dysfunction, however it is extremely rare and would be less likely to respond well to L-DOPA therapy (as this man has).

20. Arrhythmias

C. A form of ventricular tachycardia that can self-correct but can also lead to sudden death

Torsades de pointes is a rare form of ventricular tachycardia. If a new waveform was drawn by joining up the peaks and troughs, it would look roughly sinusoidal. The name derives from the sense that appears as if a normal electrocardiogram (ECG) were rotating in time around the isoelectric baseline (i.e. rising out of the page with positive amplitude, rotating toward the reader and falling back in with negative amplitude). The expression was first coined in 1966 by Francois Dessertenne. Torsades de pointes is significant in that it can both lower arterial blood pressure (leading to syncope) and is a precursor to ventricular fibrillation and therefore sudden death. It can be caused by drugs such as tricyclic antidepressants and amiodarone and is also associated with long QT syndrome (a congenital condition), malnutrition and alcohol abuse. It is treated with intravenous magnesium and anti-arrhythmics.

Torsades de pointes, from French *torsades de pointes* = twisting of the points

Francois Dessertenne, contemporary French physician

21. Back pain

C. Magnetic Resonance Imaging (MRI) of the lumbar spine

This man is presenting with advanced signs of spinal cord compression. Initially this may present with sensory deficit and weakness, and progress to bladder and bowel disturbance. Spinal cord compression needs to be considered in any patient presenting with acute back pain, but a higher index of suspicion is required in patients with known malignancy as metastases to the spine may be a cause. Spinal cord compression is an emergency that requires prompt diagnosis to prevent lasting deficit and therefore an urgent MRI is appropriate to visualise the lesion and extent of compression. MRI is a better medium than CT scan as it allows better visualisation of the soft tissues of the spinal cord. Treatment will depend on the cause but may include urgent referral for neurosurgery.

22. Bruising in children

A. Acute lymphoblastic leukaemia

Acute lymphoblastic leukaemia (ALL) is the most common leukaemia in children and is caused by the abnormal clonal proliferation of lymphoid precursor (blast) cells that have been arrested at an early stage of development. The blast cells infiltrate the marrow and lymphoid tissue causing pancytopenia and lymphadenopathy, respectively. ALL is commonest in childhood with peak incidence at 3–4 years. The central nervous system can also be affected causing headache, vomiting, meningism, cranial nerve palsies and seizure. The marrow failure and subsequent pancytopenia produces the common features of anaemia, bleeding/bruising and infection. Bone pain is another common presenting symptom. A full blood count confirms anaemia and thrombocytopenia, but demonstrates a high white cell count (due to circulating blast cells). The investigation of choice is bone marrow aspiration, which shows a hypercellular marrow with >20% blast cells. Lumbar puncture is often also necessary in the initial setting to detect cerebral involvement. Treatment is supportive with measures (such as transfusion and antibiotics) and with chemotherapy. Chemotherapy is traditionally delivered in three main stages: remission induction, consolidation and maintenance, which can be for a number of years. Since patients with ALL are at high risk of neurological disease they are often given central nervous system prophylaxis in the form of intrathecal methotrexate and radiotherapy. The prognosis of ALL is good with appropriate treatment and 95% of children can be expected to achieve remission.

23. Management of skin lesions (2)

B. Oral aciclovir

This patient has herpes zoster infection. Herpes zoster is caused by the varicella zoster virus, which is responsible for chickenpox. After an episode of chickenpox, the virus resides in dorsal root ganglia and can be transported retrogradely along the sensory axons to emerge and cause herpes zoster, most commonly in a dermatomal distribution (although it can be diffuse, usually in immunosuppressed patients). It appears most commonly on the trunk and is called "shingles", however it can affect branches of the trigeminal nerve, most commonly the ophthalmic, where it can also cause conjunctivitis, keratitis or iridocyclitis. Concurrent illness or immunosuppression can trigger zoster, and it is more common in the elderly. Many episodes will resolve spontaneously after around 2 weeks so the decision to treat depends on severity. Oral aciclovir is usually the first port of call, although intravenous aciclovir can be used in disseminated zoster. Topical acyclovir or steroids are unlikely to help, and topical antibiotics are not indicated unless there is concurrent bacterial infection.

Varicella, from Latin *variola* = spotted

Herpes, from Greek *herpein* = to crawl

Zoster, from Greek *zoster* = a belt or zone

24. Coarctation of the aorta

B. Electrocardiogram

Coarctation of the aorta is accurately diagnosed by magnetic resonance angiography. An ECG does not normally show any diagnostic changes. Collateral vessels may be visible around the scapulae. Upper limb pulses are stronger than lower limb pulses and this can be an indicator of coarctation in the absence of peripheral vascular disease (unlikely in a 14-year-old) but only if the brachial artery assessed is proximal to the coarctation. The coarctation may reside between the right brachiocephalic artery and the left subclavian artery leading to radial pulse asymmetry, or distal to them both leading to radio-femoral delay. A reduced ankle brachial pressure index may also be present.

25. Management of asthma (2)

A. Add inhaled long-acting beta-2 agonist

The pharmacological management of chronic asthma follows a stepwise approach. There are five steps in the management. In step 1, patients with mild intermittent asthma are prescribed an inhaled short-acting beta-2 agonist. If there has been an exacerbation of asthma in the last 2 years, if patient uses inhaled beta-2 agonists three times a week or more, or if patient reports symptoms three times a week or more, then inhaled corticosteroids should be added on. In step 3, if the patient's asthma control remains poor, an add-on therapy should be considered such as a long-acting beta-2 agonist. If the long-acting beta-2 agonist is not working, addition of other therapies such as leukotriene receptor antagonists or theophylline can be considered. In step 4, the inhaled corticosteroid can be increased to 2000 µg/day as well as the addition of a fourth drug (e.g. leukotriene receptor antagonist, theophylline) if symptoms persist. The final step involves continuous or frequent use of oral prednisolone. Osteoporosis can be prevented by using bisphosphonates. Once asthma control is established, the dose of the inhaled or oral corticosteroid should be titrated to the lowest dose at which effective control can be achieved.

26. Collapse (2)

B. Adrenal insufficiency

Hyponatraemia and hyperkalaemia in a patient presenting with postural hypotension indicates a possible diagnosis of primary adrenal insufficiency (Addison's disease). Adrenal insufficiency results in an inadequate secretion of cortisol and/or aldosterone. Features of an acute adrenal crisis include hyponatraemia, hyperkalaemia and circulatory shock with severe hypotension. There may be unexplained pyrexia, nausea and vomiting, diarrhoea, and muscle cramps.

To diagnose adrenal insufficiency the short synacthen test is used. Synacthen, a synthetic adrenocorticotropic hormone (ACTH) analogue, is given to the patient and the cortisol response is noted. In normal individuals, synacthen will stimulate the adrenal cortex to secrete cortisol. In patients with adrenal insufficiency, the cortex is unable to respond and the cortisol levels remain low. A cortisol level of >550 nmol/L 30 minutes after synacthen administration excludes adrenal insufficiency. If the result is positive or equivocal the patient should have a long synacthen test. In this investigation cortisol is measured at 1, 4, 8 and 24 hours after synacthen administration. In primary adrenal insufficiency (Addison's disease) the cortisol will never exceed 550 nmol/L. If the insufficiency is caused by corticotrophin-releasing hormone (CRH) or ACTH deficiency, it is termed "secondary adrenal deficiency". In secondary adrenal insufficiency the cortisol level is likely to surpass 550 nmol/L but the response is delayed.

27. Diagnosis of abdominal pain (2)

E. Spontaneous bacterial peritonitis (SBP)

Patients with ascites are at risk of developing SBP, which usually presents with severe generalised abdominal pain, worsening ascites, vomiting, fever and rigors. The most common causative organisms are Gram-negative bacilli such as *Escherichia coli* and *Klebsiella* spp., which enter the systemic circulation from the intestinal lumen and colonise the ascitic fluid. SBP can lead to rapid decompensation of liver disease causing hepatic encephalopathy and death. The diagnosis of SBP is confirmed by paracentesis, which involves taking a sample of ascitic fluid from the abdomen using a needle. The aspirated ascitic fluid is analysed for white cell count, glucose and protein. In addition, the fluid should be sent to microbiology for culture and Gram staining. If the white cell count is above 250 cells/mm³ the patient requires intravenous antibiotics (e.g. cefotaxime or ceftriaxone). Some patients also require human albumin solution to restore their intravascular fluid volume. Patients who have had a previous episode of SBP, and patients who are considered to be at high risk of developing SBP, should be considered for prophylactic oral antibiotics (e.g. norfloxacin or ciprofloxacin). The development of spontaneous bacterial peritonitis corresponds to a poor long-term prognosis.

28. Investigation of stroke

A. Carotid Doppler

The carotid Doppler is unlikely to be helpful as the infarct was clearly in the posterior circulation territory. The ECG may reveal atrial fibrillation, which is especially a possibility given his hyperthyroidism. As he is quite young for a stroke, it is important to be aware of unusual causes; a full blood count (FBC) may reveal polycythaemia (he is a smoker in his 50s) or an abnormal platelet reading, and the ESR may be elevated if there is a vasculitic process behind the infarct – he has a background of autoimmune disease. Magnetic resonance angiography (MRA) will show if there is an obvious site of posterior circulation occlusion, and in the absence of any obvious reason, this may be helpful in guiding further investigation and management, e.g. intravenous angiography +/– stenting for vertebral artery dissection.

29. Diagnosis of cough (2)

C. Sarcoidosis

Sarcoidosis is a multisystem granulomatous disease of unknown cause. It commonly affects adults aged 20–40 years old. Afro-Caribbean individuals are affected more frequently and more severely than Caucasians, particularly having extrathoracic disease. Around 20–40% of patients are asymptomatic and it is discovered incidentally on chest X-ray. Of patients with a pulmonary component of sarcoidosis, 90% have an abnormal chest X-ray with bilateral hilar lymphadenopathy with or without pulmonary infiltrates or fibrosis. Symptoms include dry cough, progressive dyspnoea, reduced exercise tolerance and chest pain. Other features include erythema nodosum (painful, purple, tender lesions on the shins), lupus pernio (sarcoidosis lesions on the skin), arthralgia and lymphadenopathy. Sarcoid tissue can activate vitamin D and cause hypercalcaemia.

Serum calcium and angiotensin-converting enzyme (ACE) levels are elevated and the tuberculin test is negative. The diagnosis of sarcoidosis is confirmed by biopsy and histology (showing non-caseating granulomas). The Kveim–Siltzbach test – where a sample of splenic tissue is injected into the skin in order to try and produce granulation tissue – is no longer done. Sarcoidosis is staged according to chest X-ray findings as follows:

Stage 1: bilateral hilar lymphadenopathy
Stage 2: bilateral hilar lymphadenopathy and lung involvement

Stage 3: lung involvement only
Stage 4: lung fibrosis

Treatment is with steroids and immunosupressants.

Sarcoid, from Greek *sark* = flesh (+ -oid) i.e. flesh-like. Describing the granulomatous deposition seen in the disease

Morton Ansgar Kveim, Norwegian pathologist (1892-1966)

Louis Siltzbach, American physician (1906-1980)

30. Diagnosis of multiple sclerosis (2)

B. Oligoclonal bands on electrophoresis

Whilst there is sometimes a rise in lymphocytes, this is both mild and rare, and given the pathology you might not expect to see red blood cells in the cerebrospinal fluid, which is backed up by observation. The protein level can be elevated, but this is rather non-specific. Whilst no single specific antigen has been identified in multiple sclerosis, antibodies to various myelinating cell-associated proteins have been found in patients with multiple sclerosis, myelin basic protein among them. However, testing for this autoantibody alone would not be sensitive enough. Oligoclonal bands on electrophoresis are found in 50–60% of patients after the first attack, and up to 95% of patients with established disease. Whilst this isn't entirely MS specific, being found in chronic meningitis, neurosarcoidosis and rare infectious nervous system diseases, they persist indefinitely in MS unlike the other disorders, and when combined with an appropriate clinical picture are highly suggestive of multiple sclerosis.

31. Investigation of abdominal pain

D. Hepatic vein Doppler ultrasound scan (USS)

Sudden-onset ascites with tender hepatomegaly in the absence of jaundice should hold a high degree of suspicion for Budd–Chiari syndrome. This syndrome describes the effects of hepatic vein outflow obstruction, commonly by thrombosis or malignant obstruction. Risk factors include malignancy, thrombophilias, trauma and the oral contraceptive pill. This can present either acutely or chronically. Diagnosis is made by Doppler scanning of the hepatic vein or venography. A similar clinical picture is produced by right-sided heart failure, constrictive pericarditis and inferior vena cava obstruction, which should also be excluded during your investigations. Treatment depends on the cause but may involve thrombolysis.

George Budd, English physician (1808-1882)

Hans Chiari, Austrian pathologist (1851-1916)

32. Diagnosis of cough (3)

D. Tuberculosis

Tuberculosis (TB) is the most common infection in the world, with a greater risk in developing countries, HIV infection and malnutrition. Although the incidence of tuberculosis in northwestern Europe and North America has declined in the latter half of the twentieth century, case rates have increased over the past 10 years secondary to immigration, the spread of HIV/AIDS, and the neglect of tuberculosis-control programmes. It is caused by the Gram-positive organism *Mycobacterium tuberculosis*, although some cases are caused by *M. bovis* and *M. africanum*. Primary TB infection occurs through droplet infection and to the development of the primary lung lesion (a focus of TB organisms surrounded by macrophages, known as the Ghon focus). This may be associated with enlarged hilar lymph nodes (Ghon complex), but is often asymptomatic. The pathology of TB is caseating granulomas. Spontaenous healing occurs in 90% of primary lesions, although a severe, disseminated infection occurs in 10% (miliary TB – seen as 1–2 mm fine lesions through the lung fields on X-ray). Re-infection or reactivation of TB results in postprimary disease. Post-primary pulmonary TB presents with a subacute illness with cough, haemoptysis, dyspnoea, fever, night sweats and anorexia. A chest X-ray shows lesions in the upper lobes. Features of extrapulmonary TB include painless lymphadenopathy, constrictive pericarditis, ascites, spinal disease, septic arthritis and kidney infection.

The diagnosis of TB can be made by sputum staining (using Ziehl–Neelsen stain) and culture (on Lowenstein–Jensen media; this can take up to 6 weeks). The bacille Calmette–Guerin (bCG) vaccine is made of attenuated *M. bovis* and provides some protection. Skin tuberculin testing can be used to screen for TB. There are two types: the Heaf test (a multipuncture method that is read after 5 days and is positive if there is ring-shaped induration) and the Mantoux test (an intradermal tuberculin injection that is read at 3 days and is positive when induration is >5 mm). False negatives to tuberculin screening are seen with severe TB, human immunodeficiency virus (HIV), malnutrition, malignancy and sarcoidosis and in people taking immunosuppressants. Drug treatment of TB is with 6 months of antituberculous therapy (e.g. rifampicin, isoniazid, pyrazinamide and ethambutol for 4 months followed by just rifampicin and isoniazid for 2 months). Ethambutol can be omitted if drug resistance is unlikely (e.g. in white, HIV-negative patients). Treatment is given for 12 months for central nervous system disease. Multidrug-resistant TB (MDRTB) is defined as TB infection that is resistant to rifampicin and isoniazid.

MRDTB is treated with five drugs for 24 months (including e.g. clarithromycin and streptomycin). Drugs are given as a single daily dose before breakfast.

The side effects of the commonly used antituberculous drugs are as follows:

- Rifampicin: orange urine, purple tears, hepatitis, induced liver enzymes
- Isoniazid: hepatitis, peripheral neuropathy
- Pyrazinamide: hepatitis, photosensitivity, gout
- Ethambutol: optic neuritis
- Streptomycin: ototoxic, nephrotoxic

Anton Ghon, Austrian pathologist (1866-1936)

Miliary, from Latin *miliarius* = grain seeds

33. Diagnosis of tuberculosis

D. Perihilar ground-glass changes

A cavitating lesion is not the most common appearance of tuberculosis on chest X-ray but it could represent a tuberculoma; it could also be a tumour, abscess or granuloma. Lobar consolidation can be seen and has a differential of bacterial pneumonia (although the symptoms and their length differentiate this). The diffuse small opacifications sounds like miliary tuberculosis, which suggests a blood-borne dissemination that will usually be more acute in onset and tuberculosis may be affecting other organs. Tuberculosis can cause pleural effusions, however, the perihilar ground-glass change does not suggest tuberculosis. Hilar lymphadenopathy can be seen in tuberculosis. Finally, tuberculosis is diagnosed when the mycobacteria are seen and multiple sputum samples should be sent for staining and culture. The absence of classical X-ray changes does not rule it out.

34. Thrombocytopenia

D. Heparin-induced thrombocytopenia (HIT)

Thrombocytopenia can be induced by a number of drugs. Low-molecular-weight heparin (LMWH) is commonly prescribed in hospital for the prevention and treatment of deep vein thrombosis and pulmonary embolism. Side effects of heparin on platelets are a relatively common idiosyncratic reaction, although there is a markedly reduced incidence when using LMWH compared to intravenous unfractionated heparin. In HIT, the platelet count reduces around 5 to 14 days after the initial exposure. There are two types:

1. Type 1 HIT is a non-immune transient asymptomatic thrombocytopenia that is seen in up to 10% of patients given heparin. Platelet levels usually remain above 80×10^9/ml and no treatment is required. The platelet count improves spontaneously even when heparin is continued.
2. Type 2 HIT is a rare but serious condition that may result in multi-organ failure and death secondary to an autoimmune process. It is caused by an immune reaction against the complex of heparin and platelet factor 4.

These complexes are removed from the circulation, resulting in thrombocytopenia. However, in doing so the release of platelet factor 4 into the circulation causes the activation of the remaining platelets. This leads to the situation of coexistent thrombocytopenia and thrombosis (arterial and venous). Type 2 HIT is seen in approximately 3–5% of patients who are prescribed unfractionated heparin but is much less common with LMWH. If Type 2 HIT is suspected, heparin must be stopped immediately and an alternative treatment instigated. Thrombolytic agents such as streptokinase may be needed to treat significant thrombosis.

Evans syndrome is an autoimmune disease against red cells and platelets, resulting in an autoimmune haemolytic anaemia and thrombocytopenia

35. Meningitis

C. Pneumococcal meningitis

The sudden onset and severe nature with sepsis precludes viral meningitis. There seems to be no overt risk of immunocompromise (homelessness, promiscuity or intravenous drug use) and the onset was acute, thus making tubercular meningitis unlikely. The lack of likely immunocompromise, age below 50 and lack of cranial nerve involvement all point away from *Listeria* meningitis. Given the alcoholism and recent chest infection, pneumococcal meningitis seems quite likely and carries a worse prognosis than meningococcal meningitis – a 20% mortality rather than 10% in meningococcal disease. His low GCS and sepsis (fever, tachycardia and low blood pressure) are also bad signs and this man may require intensive care unit (ITU) admission.

Meningitis, from Greek *menix* = membrane

36. Electrocardiogram (2)

A. Hyperkalaemia

The T-wave on an ECG denotes the repolarisation of the myocardium after systole. In the context of a patient presenting with chest pain, an inverted T-wave is a sign of myocardial infarction (also indicated by ST elevation/depression and the development of Q-waves). A similar process, to a lesser degree, occurs in myocardial ischaemia. Left ventricular hypertrophy and left bundle branch block change the nature of ventricular myocardium repolarised and hence may also invert the T-wave. Hyperkalaemia will increase the rate of repolarisation that leads to a peaked or "tented" T-wave, rather than an inverted one. The accompanying P-wave may reduce and the QRS complex may broaden. Hyperkalaemia is potentially serious and may lead to asystole or ventricular fibrillation. Hypokalaemia may flatten the T-wave and yield subtle U-waves (downward deflections) after the T-wave.

Hypokalaemia may lead to cardiac arrhythmias, constipation and fatigue, and is commonly caused by diuretics.

37. Diarrhoea (2)

E. Overflow diarrhoea

Constipation is common and can be a very debilitating condition in the elderly population. It can present with pain and discomfort and is more common in people who are immobile for long periods of time or on multiple painkillers. Spurious diarrhoea such as described can occur as watery stool manages to escape around the impacted faeces, often giving a mixed picture of diarrhoea on the background of constipation. Treatment for constipation begins with lifestyle, increasing the amount of fluid drunk, encouraging mobilisation where possible and withholding or changing constipating drugs such as opiates. Pharmacological treatments include osmotic laxatives such as lactulose, which draw water into the stool, a bulk-forming laxative such as bran, and stimulant laxatives such as movicol or glycerine suppositories.

38. Management of epilepsy

D. Valproate may cause gum hypertrophy

Even when medicated, it is a Driver and Vehicle Licensing Agency (DVLA) regulation that patients abstain from driving for 1 year after their last attack. That is, unless they have had seizures only in their sleep for the last 3 years. Whilst the patient is under 25 years, the focal nature of the attack onset is an indication for a CT/MRI to look for a structural cause, e.g. tumour or arterio-venous malformation. Valproate can cause hair loss, thrombocytopenia and hepatitis, but gum hypertrophy is not a common side effect – it is a side effect of phenytoin.

39. Diagnosis of HIV-related illness

A. Bronchoalveolar lavage

Pneumocystis pneumonia is the commonest AIDS-defining illness, caused by the fungus *Pneumocystis jiroveci* (previously known as *Pneumocystis carinii*). Patients present with a dry cough, fever, shortness of breath, weight loss and night sweats.

Bronchoalveolar lavage involves bronchoscopy and thus is quite invasive, but it is highly sensitive and 90% specific (95% with biopsy). Radiological changes can be conspicuously absent early on, but a perihilar ground-glass pattern of change can be found. Sputum cytology on sputum obtained by hypertonic saline nebuliser induction is specific although less sensitive than bronchoalveolar lavage – as low as 30% sensitive. Hypoxaemia on the arterial blood gas is a non-specific finding. The other advantage of bronchoalveolar lavage is that it will be specific in the diagnosis of other HIV-related pulmonary diseases such as tuberculosis.

Treatment is with co-trimoxazole (trimethoprim and sulphamethoxazole). Patients with HIV who have a low CD4 count ($<200/\mu l$) receive prophylaxis for pneumocystis (e.g. co-trimoxazole or dapsone).

40. Tiredness

E. Vitamin B$_{12}$ deficiency

This pattern of symptoms represent the complications of vitamin B$_{12}$ deficiency: a macrocytic anaemia, glossitis and peripheral neuropathy. Vitamin B$_{12}$ is an essential water-soluble vitamin required for DNA synthesis and red blood cell production. Vitamin B$_{12}$ is absorbed in the terminal ileum only after binding intrinsic factor, which is secreted by gastric parietal cells. The liver is able to store approximately 1 mg of vitamin B$_{12}$, sufficient for 3–4 years, hence B$_{12}$ deficiency takes years to manifest. The main causes of vitamin B$_{12}$ deficiency are pernicious anaemia (commonest in the UK), poor dietary intake (vegans) and malabsorption secondary to disease of the terminal ileum. Pernicious anaemia describes the autoimmune loss of parietal cells and/or intrinsic factor, thus preventing the absorption of vitamin B$_{12}$. It is commonest in women over 60 years. Around 90% of patients demonstrate anti-parietal antibodies (but some normal women also have it) and 60% are found to have anti-intrinsic factor antibody (which is a more specific marker).

Patients with bowel pathology, such as Crohn's disease, have normal levels of intrinsic factor but cannot absorb the B$_{12}$-intrinsic factor complex due to disease of the terminal ileum. Although most patents with pernicious anaemia complain of lethargy and general malaise, specific features of vitamin B$_{12}$ deficiency include peripheral neuropathy, smooth tongue, angular stomatitis, depression, dementia and subacute degeneration of the spinal cord. The blood film is likely to show a macrocytic ($\uparrow$MCV), megaloblastic anaemia with hypersegmented neutrophil nuclei (>6 lobes). In addition, serum vitamin B$_{12}$ levels are low and ferritin levels are normal, reflecting normal iron stores. The two-part Schilling test distinguishes pernicious anaemia from intestinal causes of B$_{12}$ deficiency – look it up if you're feeling keen! Treatment is with hydroxocobalamin (an intramuscular preparation of vitamin B$_{12}$), which is given as a 1 mg dose every other day until the blood film and symptoms improve, followed by 1 mg injections every 3 months.

The term "megaloblast" describes an abnormally large nucleated erythrocyte precursor found in people deficient in B$_{12}$ or folate

41. Management of acne (1)

C. Most people feel depressed on isotretinoin

Isotretinoin is a vitamin A analogue that markedly reduces the production of sebum. Increased sebum production is believed to contribute to the pathogenesis of acne vulgaris, as hair follicles blocked off with hyperkeratosis, which subsequently have raised sebum production within, become comedones, and it is here that the conditions are rife for *Proprionibacterium acnes* to proliferate and induce an inflammatory response. When other therapies have failed, when lesions are severe, when scarring is beginning to form or a patient is psychologically affected, systemic isotretinoin can be used, and it leads to complete clearance in 90% of patients. Dry lips is an extremely common side effect and other skin areas can become very dry – this is the mode of action of the drug so the patient must attempt to put up with as much as possible rather than cover the dry skin in thick moisturisers. Isotretinoin is highly teratogenic and therefore with female patients of reproductive age, a frank discussion should be held regarding contraception. Hyperlipidaemia and raised liver function tests are common and should be monitored – they often resolve after termination of therapy.

There are some reports of an increased incidence of depression amongst patients taking isotretinoin, although these are not consistently reproduced, and the return of someone's skin to a normal appearance can often ameliorate depression rather than cause it. Patients should be warned that there is a concern that some patients might become depressed when on isotretinoin and to be vigilant for this, but not that most people feel depressed as this is untrue.

Acne, from Latin *acne* = eruption

42. Epigastric pain (2)

E. Upper gastrointestinal (GI) endoscopy

Gastric cancer can have a devastating prognosis as it is a silent cancer that generally presents late. Signs and symptoms are often vague, with epigastric pain in people with a previous history of reflux disease or peptic ulcer disease. Adenocarcinoma is the most common type. Endoscopy is the investigation of choice as it allows for a tissue diagnosis and histology, with CT being a supplementary study to determine stage and metastases. Treatment for early gastric cancers or for palliative reasons is with surgery. The 5-year survival for all grades is 30–40%.

43. Sexually transmitted infections (1)

C. His partners should be tested for *Chlamydia* and treated with antibiotics regardless of outcome

In chlamydial infection, symptoms may be absent or mild and can resolve spontaneously. The patient will remain infectious for several months, however, and there is a risk of developing epididymo-orchitis or Reiter's syndrome (urethritis, seronegative arthritis and conjunctivitis). Regarding his partners, 80% of females are asymptomatic with chlamydial infection, laboratory tests are not 100% sensitive, and again, while infection may spontaneously resolve, others may progress to pelvic inflammatory disease and tubal damage with risk of infertility or ectopic pregnancy. Therefore, antibiotics should be given to all partners. Testing should be offered as well despite the need for antibiotics regardless of outcome, as positive tests can guide further contact tracing.

Hans Conrad Reiter, German military physician (1881-1969)

44. Non-steroidal anti-inflammatories

C. Concomitant steroid use

NSAIDs can cause bronchospasm and therefore should be avoided in asthma. NSAIDs commonly cause gastric erosions and ulceration and therefore should be avoided in aspirin users due to the risk of severe gastrointestinal bleeding; for the same reason they should be avoided when there is a significant history of gastric or duodenal ulcers. Anyone taking long-term NSAIDs should be considered for use of a proton pump inhibitor. NSAIDs can cause fluid retention and so should be avoided in patients with moderate or severe heart failure. In diseases such as rheumatoid arthritis, NSAIDs and steroids are commonly used together.

45. Renal transplantation

B. High-pressure urinary tract, e.g. posterior urethral valves

Active or chronic infection is a contraindication, as the required immunosuppression could lead to extreme worsening of infection, and the transplant could become infected or the patient could die. Malignancy not only could spread to the transplant, but it could become worse with immunosuppression and the patient is also likely to have a shortened life expectancy. If the iliac vessels are stenosed, the transplanted kidney is unlikely to be perfused well enough to function properly (given that the blood supply to the transplant comes from the iliac vessels). Severe ischaemic heart disease is a contraindication to renal transplantation.

Posterior urethral valves can affect male newborns, and can be mild or severe in their obstruction of the urinary tract. Without timely intervention, the urinary tract (including the bladder) can become high pressure and the kidneys can fail. Transplanting a new kidney onto a high-pressure tract is likely to accelerate failure of the transplant. This needn't prevent transplant and, if it is a severe problem, an ileal conduit or neobladder can be formed as an alternative to the high-pressure tract.

46. Thrombolysis in stroke

C. 2 hours post onset, BP 160/95 mmHg, GCS 15, MRI shows infarct

Thrombolysis has been proven to decrease death and severe disability if given within 3 hours of the onset of symptoms in ischaemic stroke. Some centres have started treating within 6 hours of symptom onset, so the patient who presented 7 hours after onset is ineligible. Blood pressure above 180/110 mmHg conveys too high a risk of haemorrhage post thrombolysis. Thrombolysis is obviously contraindicated by anything on a brain scan suggesting haemorrhage. A low Glasgow Coma score also precludes thrombolytic treatment, which leaves patient C.

47. Diagnosis of chest pain (2)

A. Acute pericarditis

The acute pericarditis, secondary to a viral infection, has caused these symptoms. In addition, heart sounds may be soft, indicating a pericardial effusion is underway. A chest X-ray could confirm this by demonstrating a globular heart. Cardiac tamponade is usually caused by a penetrating wound to the heart, causing haemorrhage into the pericardium. As the fibrous pericardium is inelastic, the bleed reduces the room into which the diastolic heart can expand and this, in turn, reduces cardiac output and may well be fatal. It can be treated by puncturing the pericardium with a large-bore needle to allow relief of the pressure. Whilst the needle is inserted, it should be kept in contact with an ECG lead; the live trace will jump when the needle reaches the myocardium (too far). Pulmonary embolus is a possible diagnosis for this woman but is less likely given the ECG findings.

48. Management of oliguria (2)

B. Flush the catheter with 50 ml warm saline and then aspirate

The problem that seems to have occurred here, and is quick and easy to diagnose, is that clots of blood may be being retained and blocking the end of the catheter (clot retention). Flushing the catheter with some warm saline and then aspirating may dislodge the clot and allow some urine and smaller clots to pass through the catheter. It may also allow the larger clot to pass through or disrupt it and allow its fragments to pass through. If this needs to be done repeatedly, a large-bore three-way catheter (with a separate channel for irrigation) can be inserted. Removing the catheter alone is unlikely to resolve the fact that clots are blocking the urinary tract. Insertion of a suprapubic catheter seems unnecessary at this stage and is associated with a high morbidity, due to potential perforation of the bowel, and severe urinary tract infections can occur. Requesting an ultrasound of the urinary tract would be superfluous at this stage, as clinically there is a likely cause (a large bladder is felt and there is a history of macroscopic haematuria). The patient may indeed be slightly dry, but clinically this is not the most likely cause of the renal impairment. A fluid challenge could be given if an obstructive uropathy can be ruled out, to see if hypovolaemia was indeed the cause, and intravenous fluids may still be needed if the catheter can begin draining with the saline irrigation.

49. The unresponsive patient (2)

E. Subdural haematoma

The first thing to note is that it is possible that the low GCS and confusion could be due to something separate, e.g. overuse of opioids and an otherwise asymptomatic urinary tract infection (UTI) – but opioid use is likely to have been highest on admission with the pain from the injury subsequently decreasing. Action would be taken to rule out such things but as the defects have all started together, and an intracranial cause would be the most worrying explanation, an intracranial lesion must be considered. Whilst meningitis can give focal neurological defects and a decreased GCS, the stable observations, lack of a temperature, and lack of reported headache, neck stiffness or photophobia make this unlikely. A lacunar infarct can present as a pure motor weakness with no other focal defect, however, this is likely to come on acutely with decreased reflexes and there is unlikely to be a drop in GCS. Subarachnoid haemorrhage can present with a drop in GCS and focal neurology, but more commonly present with unconsciousness, seizures or thunderclap headache with meningism, which are all absent. There is no reason in the story why a subarachnoid haemorrhage would cause deficits to appear at this stage. Strokes do not usually cause a drop in GCS, although a large intracerebral haemorrhage could by mass effect – however, the neurology in the patient is subacute, mild and limited. An intracerebral haemorrhage large enough to drop the GCS would give more than simply mild motor weakness, and do so more acutely (though neurology could progress as the haemorrhage and oedema evolved).

This patient is an elderly woman who could have possibly sustained a head injury and may be an alcoholic – these factors put her at risk of a subdural haemorrhage. Subdural haemorrhage commonly presents with a subacute development of impaired GCS and focal neurology, and does not always have a history of head injury and therefore this seems the most likely explanation. In any case, a computed tomography (CT) scan of the head is indicated and would show any of the lesions discussed.

50. Thyrotoxicosis

A. Graves' disease

This is a typical picture of a person who has thyrotoxicosis in which the most common symptoms are weight loss with a normal or increased appetite, heat intolerance, palpitations, tremor and irritability. In all causes of thyrotoxicosis, the patient would present with lid lag and lid retraction. Graves' disease is the only cause of other ophthalmological symptoms such as periorbital oedema, conjunctival irritation, exophthalmos and diplopia.

Graves' disease is the commonest cause of hyperthyroidism. It is an autoimmune disease in which circulating IgG immunoglobulins stimulate the TSH receptors of the thyroid gland, causing the release of thyroxine into the circulation. Autoantibodies are also directed against retro-orbital structures causing proptosis, ophthalmoplegia and peri-orbital oedema.

Robert James Graves, Irish physician (1797-1853)

Practice Paper 3: Questions

1. Acute coronary syndrome (3)

A 55-year-old man has presented to the medical admissions unit with chest pain. You have diagnosed acute coronary syndrome (ACS) and are about to write up his drug chart.

Your most suitable prescription would be:

A 75 mg aspirin, clopidogrel, treatment dose heparin *stat* with glyceryl trinitrite (GTN) spray and morphine PRN

B 75 mg aspirin, clopidogrel, treatment dose heparin and beta-blocker *stat* with GTN spray and morphine PRN

C 300 mg aspirin, clopidogrel, prophylactic dose heparin *stat* with GTN spray and morphine PRN

D 300 mg aspirin, clopidogrel, treatment dose heparin and beta-blocker *stat* with GTN spray and morphine PRN

E 300 mg aspirin, prophylactic heparin and beta-blocker *stat* with GTN spray and morphine PRN

2. Haematuria

A 32-year-old man presents to the GP 4 days after an episode of painless haematuria, 2 weeks following a sore throat. He says he now feels he is producing less urine than usual and that it is brown. He denies any weight loss or fatigue, and has no family history of urological malignancy. On examination, he has a blood pressure of 155/90 mmHg, +++ blood on urine dipstick, and blood tests reveal a creatinine of 170 μmol/L and normal electrolytes.

What is the clinical picture most consistent with?

A Acute tubular necrosis
B Nephritic syndrome
C Nephrotic syndrome
D Renal calculi
E Transitional cell carcinoma of the bladder

3. Heart failure (2)

In the treatment of heart failure with atrial fibrillation, which of the following statements about digoxin is false?

A ACE inhibitors and beta-blockers are more effective at extending survival
B Digoxin has a secondary vagal effect that slows heart rate
C Digoxin is effective at treating the symptoms
D Digoxin is obtained from foxgloves
E Digoxin is primarily a chronotropic drug

4. Hodgkin's lymphoma

A 32-year-old man is diagnosed with Hodgkin's lymphoma following a recent history of weight loss and night sweats. Computed tomography (CT) staging scan shows disease in the mediastinum bilaterally and some abdominal lymphadenopathy, including the spleen, but no evidence of disease in extranodal sites.

What is his stage of disease?

A Stage IIA
B Stage IIB
C Stage IIIA
D Stage IIIB
E Stage IVB

5. Management of psoriasis

A 35-year-old woman with a 1-year history of plaque psoriasis is having difficulty with management. Along with emollients, she has tried tar and dithranol, which she did not get on well with (due to the smell and burning, respectively), and has been using a combination of vitamin D analogues and Betnovate™, a potent topical steroid. She has difficulty finding time with her lifestyle to apply the creams often enough and as a result the lesions have become more widespread and she is now extremely concerned about her appearance, both in the workplace and at her sister's wedding, which is coming up soon.

Which of the following would be the best treatment to try next?

A Ciclosporin
B Infliximab
C Methotrexate
D Prednisolone
E Ultraviolet therapy

6. Subarachnoid haemorrhage

Which of the following statements about subarachnoid haemorrhage is NOT true?

A Focal weakness may ensue

B Lumbar puncture (LP) immediately on admission is likely to show xanthochromia

C Subarachnoid haemorrhage may present as a new onset of seizures

D Subarachnoid haemorrhages may be provoked by exertion or coitus

E Unenhanced CT within 48 hours is 95% sensitive

7. Overdose and antidotes (1)

A 32-year-old woman presents to the emergency department having reportedly taken a large dose of heroin. She is unresponsive, has small pupils and has a respiratory rate of 6 breaths/min.

Which of the following should be administered?

A Atropine

B Ethanol

C Flumazenil

D N-acetylcysteine

E Naloxone

8. Pneumonia

A 44-year-old man presents to the emergency department with a 3-day history of shortness of breath and a productive cough. His observations include temperature 38.2°C, pulse rate 90 bpm, blood pressure 130/86 mmHg, respiratory rate 24/min and saturations 94% on room air. Blood results include white cell count of 13.5×10^6/L, CRP 45 mmol/L, Na$^+$136 mmol/L, K$^+$4.3 mmol/L, urea 9.2 mmol/L and creatinine 110 μmol/L. On examination, he appears to be alert, and there are dull sounds on percussion over the right lower lobe. A chest X-ray confirms a right lower lung lobe consolidation.

What is the most appropriate management?

A Admission into hospital with empirical antibiotic treatment

B Admission into hospital for nebulised salbutamol and empirical antibiotic treatment

C Admission into intensive care unit

D Home with inhaled salbutamol when clinically stable

E Home with empirical antibiotic treatment when clinically stable

9. Murmur (1)

A 68-year-old obese woman is not coping at home and presents to the emergency department following a fall. On examination, she has a weak,

regular pulse and an ejection systolic murmur. You try to lean her forward and palpate her apex beat in expiration but she gets flustered and complains of a sore back and shortness of breath. A neurological examination is unremarkable and her haemoglobin level is 13.2 g/dl.

What is most likely wrong with her?

A Aortic stenosis
B Atrial fibrillation
C Cerebrovascular accident
D Gastrointestinal bleed
E Mitral regurgitation

10. Skin lesions (3)

A 70-year-old man presents with multiple widespread tense blisters measuring between 0.5 cm and 5 cm in diameter. They are localised mainly to the arms and legs, with some lesions on the chest. They appeared over weeks, preceded by itchy urticarial lesions. A few lesions have burst and have left not much behind. There is a history of osteoarthritis of the knees for which he takes diclofenac, and he has not changed any medication in the past year. A subsequent biopsy of a bulla shows splitting at the dermoepidermal junction.

What is the diagnosis?

A Insect bites
B Pemphigoid
C Pemphigus
D Stevens–Johnson syndrome
E Toxic epidermal necrolysis

11. Antibiotics (2)

Which of the following antibiotic and side-effect pairings is FALSE?

A Ceftriaxone and tendon rupture
B Co-amoxiclav and cholestatic jaundice
C Erythromycin and diarrhoea
D Gentamicin and nephrotoxicity
E Nitrofurantoin and pulmonary fibrosis

12. Scoring systems (2)

Which of the following scoring systems should be used to assess a patient's risk of developing a pressure score?

A Breslow score
B Confusion, Urea, Respiratory rate, Blood pressure, Age (CURB) score
C Ranson's criteria
D Rockall score
E Waterlow score

13. Investigation of headache (2)

A 78-year-old woman, who has recently been feeling under the weather and losing some weight, develops a severe left-sided headache with jaw pain on eating. She also complains of blurred vision on the left side.

Which of the following investigations is needed to give a definitive diagnosis?

A Computed tomography (CT) of the head
B Erythrocyte sedimentation rate (ESR)
C Magnetic resonance imaging (MRI) of the head
D Temporal artery biopsy
E Ultrasound of the temporal arteries

14. Management of hyperglycaemia (1)

A 48-year-old man presents to the emergency department in a reduced state of consciousness. He was brought in by his son, who says he has been more confused over the past few days. A collateral history suggests 2 weeks of polyuria and polydipsia. There was no history of head injury, trauma or ingestion of illegal drugs. He has no other significant past medical history. He has a 21 U/week alcohol history. On examination, he is unresponsive to pain. The liver edge is felt on abdominal examination. His blood tests show:

Na^+	168 mmol/L
K^+	3.8 mmol/L
Glucose	68 mmol/L
Serum osmolality	350 mmol/kg
Urea	14.3 mmol/L
Creatinine	203 µmol/L

A urine dipstick test revealed glycosuria but no ketones.

What is the most appropriate approach to the management of this patient?

A Aim for blood glucose concentration fall by 10 mmol/L per hour
B Fluid restriction
C Give treatment dose of low-molecular-weight heparin
D Infuse 1 L of 0.9% NaCl fluid infusion with added 40 mmol potassium at a rate of 1 L/hour
E Start insulin infusion at 3 U/hour initially

15. Management of skin lesions (3)

An 81-year-old retired farmer presents with a 1.5 cm raised lesion on his left temple that has slowly grown over the past year and occasionally bleeds. He has had a basal cell carcinoma removed from his right temple previously, and he has had cryotherapy for actinic keratoses on his temples and head several times at his GP surgery. On examination, the lesion has a rolled edge and is translucent with telangiectasia.

Which of the following treatment options is NOT recommended for this lesion?

A Chemotherapy
B Excision
C Mohs micrographic surgery
D Radiotherapy
E Topical 5-fluorouracil

16. Fatigue

A 35-year-old man presents to the GP with increasing fatigue for 3 months. He finds himself waking up choking a few times at night. He was told by his partner that he snores quite loudly most nights. He denies any weight loss. He smokes 30 cigarettes/day, drinks 2 pints of beer every night and has a body mass index of 32.

What is the most likely differential diagnosis?

A Central sleep apnoea
B Chronic fatigue syndrome
C Idiopathic hypersomnolence
D Narcolepsy
E Obstructive sleep apnoea

17. Arterial blood gases (1)

A 73-year-old man has been admitted with severe sepsis and acute renal failure secondary to a urinary tract infection. He has been treated with intravenous antibiotics and fluid resuscitation but the following day you are called to see him as he is worse. He looks extremely unwell. His airway is patent and he has laboured breathing at a rate of 22 breaths/min. His saturations are 98% on air and his chest sounds clear. His pulse is 120 bpm and blood pressure 85/55 mmHg. His capillary refill rate is 4 seconds. His urine output has been 40 ml in the last 5 hours. You see from his blood tests that his creatinine level has increased slightly. You take an arterial blood gas reading.

Which of the following is the most likely result?

A pH 7.22, pO_2 8, pCO_2 8.3, HCO_3^- 24
B pH 7.22, pO_2 18, pCO_2 2.3, HCO_3^- 10
C pH 7.22, pO_2 18, pCO_2 8.3, HCO_3^- 10
D pH 7.40, pO_2 8, pCO_2 8.3, HCO_3^- 38
E pH 7.51, pO_2 18, pCO_2 2.3, HCO_3^- 24

18. Shortness of breath (3)

A 65-year-old man presents to the GP with chest pain, increasing shortness of breath and weight loss. He describes the pain as dull and worse on inhalation. He notices that he has lost 1 stone in 3 weeks. He has never smoked and has no other significant past medical history. He used to work in a shipyard. Observations include temperature 36.8°C, pulse rate 80 bpm, blood pressure 140/95 mmHg and respiratory rate 18/min. On examination, there is dullness to percussion over the left lower lung zone.

What is the most likely diagnosis?

A Bronchocarcinoma
B Mesothelioma
C Pneumoconiosis
D Pulmonary embolism
E Tuberculosis

19. Management of chest pain (1)

A 61-year-old woman presents to the walk-in clinic with a history of tight, sternal chest pain "appearing out of the blue". Such episodes have occurred at different times throughout the day and rarely last longer than a few minutes. They do not correspond to hard exercise. The patient has no cardiac history to date. Her electrocardiogram (ECG) has not detected any abnormalities and 2 days have passed since the last episode.

Which of the following is the next best step in her management?

A 24-hour ECG
B Admit to a ward
C Chest X-ray
D Echocardiogram
E Prescribe home oxygen

20. Barium enema

A 37-year-old woman is being investigated for weight loss and diarrhoea. Barium enema shows "cobble-stoning", rose thorn ulcers and colonic strictures at intermittent points throughout the colon.

What is the most likely diagnosis?

A Coeliac disease
B Colonic carcinoma
C Crohn's disease
D Inflammatory bowel disease
E Ulcerative colitis

21. Cardiovascular examination

You are asked by your registrar to see a 40-year-old woman and report back your findings. On examination, you struggle to find an apex beat although heart sounds 1 and 2 were audible with no murmur. On inspection, her electrocardiogram (ECG) is normal except for inverted P-waves.

What is the most likely reason for these findings?

A Dextrocardia
B Cardiomyopathy
C Mitral stenosis
D Myocardial ischaemia
E Pulmonary hypertension

22. Cauda equina syndrome

A 53-year-old man, who has had some lower back pain and sciatica into his right leg for the past year, presents with a 2-day history of leg weakness and severe pain.

On examination, which of the following signs does NOT make you think of cauda equina syndrome?

A Distended bladder
B Reduced anal tone
C Reduced reflexes in the ankles
D Saddle anaesthesia
E Upgoing plantars

23. Joint swelling

A 35-year-old man presents with a 3-week history of pain and swelling in the tips of his fingers. He has no history of bowel problems, recent infection or skin disease, but his brother has Crohn's disease. On examination you find several swollen, red, tender distal interphalangeal joints, and the nails have separated from the nailbed and have small pockmarks covering them. The rest of the examination is unremarkable.

Which of the following diagnoses is most likely?

A Enteropathic arthritis
B Osteoarthritis
C Psoriatic arthropathy
D Reactive arthritis
E Rheumatoid arthritis

24. Coeliac disease

Which of the following is a recognised complication of coeliac disease?

A Fistulae
B Intestinal lymphoma
C Primary sclerosing cholangitis
D Toxic megacolon
E Uveitis

25. Complications of alcoholic liver disease

You are called in the middle of the night to see a 49-year-old man with known alcoholic liver disease admitted 2 days previously. He is shaking, sweating, tachycardic, apyrexial and believes he is seeing spiders crawling across the ceiling.

What is the most likely diagnosis?

A Alcohol intoxication
B Delirium tremens
C Bacterial peritonitis
D Fulminant hepatic necrosis
E Urinary tract infection

26. Diagnosis of abdominal pain (3)

A 59-year-old woman with advanced metastatic breast cancer presents to the emergency department with severe abdominal pain. She has not opened her bowels for 7 days and feels constipated. She has also noticed that she has been passing water more frequently but has not been incontinent. On rectal examination there is no loss of anal tone and normal sensation.

What is the most likely diagnosis?

A Hypercalcaemia
B Hypocalcaemia
C Metastatic spread to the bowel
D Opiate-induced constipation
E Spinal cord compression

27. Disseminated intravascular coagulation

A 19-year-old female presents to the emergency department with a severe headache, photophobia, neck stiffness and a temperature. She is treated for bacterial meningitis with intravenous ceftriaxone. Blood cultures grow *Neisseria meningitides*. The next day, she starts bleeding from around her intravenous cannula and venepuncture sites.

Which of the following investigation results would you NOT expect in disseminated intravascular coagulation?

A Increased activated partial thromboplastin time (APTT)
B Increased fibrinogen
C Increased international normalised ratio (INR)
D Decreased haemoglobin
E Decreased platelets

28. Rectal bleeding (1)

A 67-year-old man presents with painless rectal bleeding for the past 2 months. It occurs mainly on defecation, and is bright red in the pan and on the toilet paper. A digital rectal examination is unremarkable.

What should your management be?

A Abdominal X-rays
B Review patient in 1 month to see if bleeding has stopped
C Routine bloods
D Routine outpatient appointment in 4–6 weeks
E Urgent 2-week outpatient referral

29. Diagnosis of cough (4)

A 23-year-old final year law student presents to the GP with a cough productive of foul green sputum. He also complains of breathlessness on exertion. He has had an average of five respiratory tract infections per year for the past 2 years. As a child, he could not tolerate dairy products. On examination, finger clubbing is present and there is dullness to percussion of the right upper lung zone with widespread bilateral wheeze.

What is the most probable diagnosis?

A Asthma
B Coeliac disease
C Cystic fibrosis
D Immotile cilia syndrome
E Pneumonia

30. Diagnosis of gout

A 50-year-old overweight pub landlord presents with an acutely painful swollen red hot first metatarsophalangeal joint on the left. You suspect gout.

Which of the following would confirm this on microscopy of a joint aspirate?

A Calcium pyrophosphate crystals
B Crystals of a rhomboid shape
C Crystals showing apple green birefringence under polarised light
D Crystals showing negative birefringence under polarised light
E Crystals showing positive birefringence under polarised light

31. Investigation of shortness of breath (1)

A 56-year-old man who has been recently diagnosed with sigmoid cancer and had a Hartmann's procedure is admitted to hospital with acute-onset shortness of breath. He denies any collapse or fainting. He has a past medical history of chronic obstructive pulmonary disease, hypertension, stroke and gout. His observations include temperature 37.2°C, pulse rate 106 bpm, blood pressure 110/74 mmHg, respiratory rate 25/min and saturations 87% on room air. There is no significant finding on chest examination. An electrocardiogram (ECG) shows sinus tachycardia with no ST elevation. A plain chest X-ray shows a small left pleural effusion.

Which of the following is the most appropriate diagnostic investigation?

A Magnetic resonance imaging (MRI) of the chest
B D-dimer level
C Computed tomographic pulmonary angiography
D Ventilation-perfusion scanning
E Echocardiography

32. Diagnosis of neurological dysfunction (1)

A 27-year-old woman who works in the city as an investment banker presents with difficulty walking, and a tremor in the right hand. It has come on over the last 4 days and she is now unable to get to work safely. She denies any preceding respiratory or gastrointestinal infection or any abnormal stress at work or in her personal life; however, she says that 5 months ago she had some pain and blurring in the left eye for about 10 days, but she put that down to "sinusitis", kept working, and things returned to normal. Her grandfather, who died 2 years ago, had Parkinson's disease for some time, and she is concerned that this could be the same thing. On examination, in her arms, there is normal tone, power and sensation, but there is indeed a tremor in the right hand on testing coordination, which gets worse on approaching the target, and is absent at rest. In the legs, there is normal power, but decreased light touch sensation bilaterally and a loss of vibration sense and proprioception up to the ankles.

What are you most concerned is the diagnosis?

A Acute disseminated encephalomyelitis
B Familial early-onset Parkinson disease
C Guillain–Barré syndrome
D Multiple sclerosis
E Psychogenic neurological symptoms

33. Management of multiple sclerosis

A 33-year-old woman with multiple sclerosis (MS) is having problems with painful spasms and disabling spasticity in her left leg.

Which of the following medications is most likely to help?

A Baclofen
B Lactulose
C Modafinil
D Oxybutinin
E Propanolol

34. Diagnosis of stroke

A 65-year-old woman presents to hospital with left-sided weakness of sudden onset. She is a type II diabetic, smokes 20 cigarettes/day and has high blood pressure. On examination, power in the left arm is 0 throughout although the left leg shows a power of 3 at the hip and knee and 4 at the foot. Her reflexes are reduced throughout, and sensation is absent in the arm and reduced in the leg. In the cranial nerve examination she is unable to see on her left-hand side, and the lower half of her left face is weak (she can raise her eyebrow). There is no dysphasia.

Which vascular territory is affected?

A Left anterior cerebral artery
B Right anterior cerebral artery
C Right carotid artery
D Right middle cerebral artery
E Right posterior cerebral artery

35. Diagnosis of cough (5)

A 45-year-old man presents to the GP with a 4-month history of a productive cough with exertional breathlessness. He denies haemoptysis or weight loss. He has a 20 pack/year smoking history. On examination, fine crackles are heard throughout the whole lung field.

What is most likely differential diagnosis?

A Asthma
B Chronic obstructive pulmonary disease
C Cystic fibrosis
D Idiopathic pulmonary fibrosis
E Lung cancer

42. Statistics (1)

A new blood test is being developed to help diagnose sarcoidosis. In a trial 100 patients have been tested. The trial produces 20 positive results and 80 negative results. Of the 20 positive results, 10 of them are false positives. Of the 80 negative results, 10 of them are false negatives.

What is the sensitivity of this test?

A 10%
B 25%
C 50%
D 75%
E 90%

43. Sexually transmitted infections (2)

A 34-year-old woman, who is known to be human immunodeficiency virus (HIV) positive, presents with multiple lesions on her face. The lesions are raised and shiny, non-tender and around 3 mm in diameter. They have an umbilicated centre.

What is the most likely diagnosis?

A Herpes simplex
B Kaposi sarcoma
C Molluscum contagiosum
D Scabies
E Syphilis

44. Management of shortness of breath (1)

A 49-year-old man presents to the emergency department with acute-onset right-sided pleuritic chest pain and shortness of breath. There was no associated trauma. He has a past medical history of chronic obstructive pulmonary disease, hypertension and diabetes mellitus. He smokes 40 cigarettes per day. His observations include temperature 37.2°C, pulse rate 95 bpm, blood pressure 150/92 mmHg, respiratory rate 24/min and saturations 92% on room air. A chest X-ray (CXR) shows a small rim of air (less than 2 cm) between the right lung edge and the chest wall.

Which of the following is the most appropriate first-line management?

A Admit to be observed only
B Intercostal tube drainage
C Medical pleurodesis
D Percutaneous needle aspiration
E Surgical pleurodesis

45. Signs of liver disease (1)

A 52-year-old man with a history of alcohol excess presents to his GP because he cannot fully extend his ring finger on his right hand (neither actively nor passively). Since the finger is permanently partially flexed he can no longer place his hand flat on a flat surface.

Which of the following is the most likely diagnosis?

A Asterixis
B Dupuytren contracture
C Palmar erythema
D Trigger finger
E Xanthelasma

46. Non-invasive ventilation

A 63-year-old man is admitted to the emergency department with severe dyspnoea. He is a longstanding smoker of 40 years. His observations are pulse rate 130 bpm, respiratory rate 36/min, oxygen saturation of 85% on 24% oxygen via a venturi mask and temperature 38.2°C. Chest examination reveals reduced air entry on both lungs with coarse crackles on his left lower lobe. Despite immediate maximum standard medical treatment on controlled oxygen therapy, his arterial blood gas still shows persistent acidosis with a $PaCO_2$ of 8 kPa.

Which of the following would NOT be a required inclusion criterion for non-invasive ventilation?

A Ability to protect his airway
B Home oxygen use
C Patient's wishes considered
D Potential for recovery to quality of life acceptable to the patient
E Primary diagnosis of chronic pulmonary obstructive disease

47. Systemic lupus erythematosus (1)

A 34-year-old woman with systemic lupus erythematosus (SLE) has had multiple miscarriages and now presents with a painful right swollen leg. A compression ultrasound scan confirms deep vein thrombosis.

Which blood test may now be indicated?

A Anti-phospholipid antibodies
B Clotting factors
C Haemoglobin
D Pregnancy test
E Tumour markers

48. Medications in hyperkalaemia

A 74-year-old man with a history of hypertension, ischaemic heart disease and moderate congestive cardiac failure is admitted with a urinary tract infection and has developed acute renal failure. His potassium level is noted to be 5.5 mmol/L.

Which of his following medications may be contributing to the raised serum potassium level?

A Amlodipine
B Bendroflumethiazide
C Furosemide
D Simvastatin
E Spironolactone

49. Tumour markers

A 42-year-old woman attends to her GP complaining of non-specific abdominal pain and an increasing abdominal girth. She is found to have a large mass in her right lower abdomen and ascites on transvaginal ultrasound imaging.

Which of the following tumour markers would be most useful?

A CA 125
B Ca 15-3
C Ca 19-9
D CEA
E Beta-hCG

50. Parkinson's disease

Which of the following best describes the four cardinal signs of Parkinson's disease?

A Bradykinesia, mask-like facies, rigidity, and tremor ~10–12 Hz
B Bradykinesia, micrographia, rigidity, and tremor ~3–4 Hz
C Bradykinesia, postural hypotension, rigidity, and tremor ~3–4 Hz
D Bradykinesia, postural instability, rigidity, and tremor ~3–4 Hz
E Bradykinesia, postural instability, rigidity, and tremor ~10–12 Hz

Practice Paper 3: Answers

1. Acute coronary syndrome (3)

D. 300 mg aspirin, clopidogrel, treatment dose heparin and beta-blocker *stat* with GTN spray and morphine PRN

Low-molecular-weight heparin (LMWH) is commonly administered as venous thromboembolism prophylaxis. The larger treatment dose indicated in acute coronary syndrome may be weight dependent. Heparin does not lyse clots but rather prevents them from forming or extending. Thrombolysis occurs continuously in the body; heparin merely arrests the clot-growing process enough for natural thrombolysis to triumph. In the event of haemorrhage, protamine sulphate reverses the effects of heparin.

2. Haematuria

B. Nephritic syndrome

Nephritic syndrome may be defined as a triad of haematuria (which can be microscopic or macroscopic), hypertension, and a reduction in the glomerular filtration rate. Along with the reduction in glomerular filtration rate and associated oliguria, oedema can be a feature, both peripheral and pulmonary, and proteinuria may also be present. Our patient needs to be investigated for a cause of his nephritic syndrome and referred to a renal physician. As well as routine bloods, ESR and CRP need to be tested to look for an inflammatory cause. Serum and urine should be sent for electrophoresis (to rule out myeloma), and a renal screen including complement (C3 and C4 – can be reduced in active lupus), anti-nuclear antibody, anti-neutrophil cytoplasm antibodies, anti-streptolysin-O titre (for post-streptococcal glomerulonephritis), anti-glomerular basement membrane antibodies (Goodpasture syndrome), and hepatitis serology. Urine should also be sent for 24-hour protein quantification (to look for concominant nephrotic syndrome) and microscopy (to look for casts). The most common glomerulonephritis in the western world is Berger disease, which is an IgA nephropathy. It usually affects young men after an upper respiratory tract infection. If renal impairment is ongoing, immunosuppression can be indicated.

Nephrotic syndrome is a triad of proteinuria, hypoalbuminaemia and oedema – oedema is not a clinical feature here, and proteinuria was not found. Nephrotic syndrome, however, can often occur with nephritic syndrome – both are commonly caused by glomerulonephritides – and so it should be tested for (with either a 24-hour urine protein quantification or a urine protein creatinine ratio). Renal calculi can cause haematuria but is associated with severe pain.

Acute tubular necrosis is a form of acute renal injury usually following renal ischaemia, due to dehydration, sepsis, hypotension or renal vascular disease. As such, it is common in hospital practice when pre-renal acute renal failure has not been sufficiently addressed. It can also rarely be caused by direct damage from drugs including aminoglycosides and lithium. There is no reason to believe that any of these drugs or causes of renal hypoperfusion have taken place. Haematuria and hypertension are not typical features of acute tubular necrosis.

3. Heart failure (2)

E. Digoxin is primarily a chronotropic drug

Digoxin, a cardiac glycoside extracted from the foxglove *Digitalis lanata*, is an inotrope. By blocking the sodium/potassium pump, it causes a rise in intracellular sodium which, via sodium–calcium exchange, increases the intracellular concentration of calcium and hence contractility. As a result of the increased effort of myocardial contraction, atrio-ventricular node delay is increased and heart rate is indirectly slowed.

Digoxin has been shown to relieve symptoms of heart failure without necessarily improving mortality but it is the only inotrope that does not actually increase mortality.

Digitalis, from Latin *digitalis* = finger, with reference to the German name
for foxglove, Fingerhut ("thimble")

4. Hodgkin's lymphoma

D. Stage IIIB

Hodgkin's lymphoma has a bimodal age distribution with peak incidences occurring in the third and sixth decades. Is it usually of B-cell origin and is associated with a history of glandular fever. It classically presents with asymmetrical painless lymphadenopathy usually in the form of a single rubbery lymph node in the cervical, axillary or inguinal region that may become painful after alcohol ingestion. Disease spread to the mediastinal nodes may cause dyspnoea and superior vena cava obstruction. Approximately 20% of patients suffer systemic symptoms such as weight loss, sweating, fever, pruritis and general lethargy. These are known as "B" symptoms and are associated with a worse prognosis. Diagnosis is usually based on lymph node biopsy showing pathognomonic Reed–Sternberg cells (large malignant B-cells). CT scanning is used to assess spread, and staging is by the Ann Arbor system (I=one node region involved, II=2+ ipsilateral regions, III=bilateral node involvement, IV=extranodal disease). The presence or absence of B symptoms is indicated in the staging by the suffix "A" (B symptoms absent) or "B" (B symptoms present). Early-stage disease is usually managed with radiotherapy alone. In advanced and bulky disease the combination of radiotherapy and chemotherapy is often employed. The prognosis of Hodgkin's lymphoma is usually good, with a 70% chance of cure even in late-stage disease. Increasing age indicates a poorer prognosis.

Thomas Hodgkin, British physician (1798-1866)

Ann Arbor is a city in the US state of Michigan, where the committee on Hodgkin disease staging classification met and revised the staging of lymphoma

5. Management of psoriasis

E. Ultraviolet therapy

There are a range of topical therapies available for psoriasis, and it can often take an amount of experimentation to find the right combination for each patient. Compliance with laborious application of creams is an issue and patients differ widely in their approach. Tar is an effective therapy, especially crude tar, but stickiness, messiness and smell mean that most patients do not like taking it. Dithranol is often used as first-line medication in chronic plaque psoriasis, however it can burn the skin (especially around the eyes) and can permanently stain clothes so needs to be used carefully. Potent steroids can be used, although they may induce a rebound phenomenon whereby lesions become worse than previously on stopping the topical steroids.

Ultraviolet therapy can be a useful next step in treatment for widespread psoriasis, as it can often rid a patient entirely of lesions without laborious cream application. The plaques often come back, however, at different rates and to different extents. It should not be given too many times in a person's life due to theoretical risk of skin cancers. It can result in sunburn, and so patients often start at a low dose and then increase the dose until the ultraviolet (UV) rays induce some erythema but not burn. Side effects and need for monitoring are markedly less than with use of systemic therapies such as methotrexate, prednisolone, ciclosporin and biological agents such as infliximab, and these should be withheld for severe psoriasis refractory to topical and UV therapies.

6. Subarachnoid haemorrhage

B. Lumbar puncture (LP) immediately on admission is likely to show xanthochromia

Xanthochromia describes a straw-coloured appearance of the cerebrospinal fluid in subarachnoid haemorrhages caused by the presence of haemoglobin breakdown products, and as such requires at least 6 hours before detection. LP at 12 hours is 95% sensitive when spectrophotometry is used to look for xanthochromia. Therefore LP on admission may not be likely to show xanthochromia. Focal weakness may indeed ensue, either from haematoma or from arterial constriction or occlusion 4–12 days post event – the surrounding blood clot, oedema and inflammatory factors induce vasoconstriction and further vessel inflammation, which could thus cause ischaemic brain damage. Of those making it into hospital, 10% present with new seizures. Extreme exertion and coitus may cause rupture of a cerebral aneurysm by sudden drastic increases in intracranial pressure. Unenhanced CT shows 95% of subarachnoid haemorrhages within 48 hours – blood enhances whiter than the surrounding brain matter due to the increased density of radio-opaque iron.

Xanthochromia, from Greek xanthos = yellow

7. Overdose and antidotes (1)

E. Naloxone

This patient is suffering from a morphine overdose and is exhibiting the classic features of reduced responsiveness, pinpoint pupils and respiratory depression. This is a significant and potentially life-threatening overdose that will require treatment with naloxone. Naloxone competes with opiates for the mu receptors. It should be noted that naloxone has a very strong affinity for mu receptors and can therefore rapidly induce opiate withdrawal and trigger seizures. It has been known for intravenous drug users to be extremely annoyed at medical staff for ruining their "high" with naloxone. Naloxone also has a shorter half-life compared to opiates, so repeated doses or an infusion may be required to maintain its beneficial effect.

Examples of antidotes and other medications used in overdose are:

- Antimuscarinic overdose — Physostigmine
- Aspirin overdose — Sodium bicarbonate
- Benzodiazepine overdose — Flumazenil
- Beta-blocker overdose — Atropine, glucagon
- Carbon monoxide poisoning — Oxygen
- Digoxin overdose — Digibind
- Heparin overdose — Protamine

- Iron overdose — Desferrioxamine
- Methanol overdose — Ethanol
- Paracetamol overdose — N-acetylcysteine
- Warfarin overdose — Vitamin K

8. Pneumonia

E. Home with empirical antibiotic treatment when clinically stable

Community-acquired pneumonia can present as a wide spectrum of illness from mild and self-limiting to life threatening. The CURB-65 score is used as an assessment of severity of pneumonia and helps decide the appropriate management. The recognition of mild disease with a low risk of complications enables patients to receive treatment at home, thus reducing inappropriate hospitalisation.

The CURB-65 score comprises five components:

- Confusion AMTS <8
- Urea >7 mmol/L
- Respiratory rate >30/min
- Blood pressure systolic <90 mmHg or diastolic 60 mmHg
- Age >65 years

Each feature scores one point. Patients with a CURB-65 score of 0 or 1 point could receive home treatment with oral antibiotics. Patients with a CURB-65 score of 2 could be considered to receive short-stay hospital-supervised treatment. Patients with a CURB-65 score of ≥3 should be managed in the hospital as severe pneumonia (associated with a mortality rate of 22%), and if the CURB-65 score is 4 or 5, ICU admission should be considered.

9. Murmur (1)

A. Aortic stenosis

Aortic stenosis can be a cause of shortness of breath and syncope due to reduced cardiac output. Post-fall back pain is very common and is simply due to trauma in this case. Ejection systolic murmurs are the classic sign of aortic stenosis, as blood is ejected through the narrowed valvular orifice under enough pressure to generate turbulent noise. The most common cause of aortic stenosis is age-related calcification. Congenital bicuspid aortic valves are also vulnerable to calcification (prevalence 1–2%), and many people have underdone aortic valve replacement surgery, including actors Arnold Schwarzenegger and Robin Williams. Rheumatic fever (post-streptococcal autoimmune attack of valve tissue) also increases calcification.

Aortic stenosis can also lead to heart failure, angina and Heyde syndrome (colonic angiodysplasia and lower gastrointestinal bleeding associated with aortic stenosis). In the latter case, valve stenosis leads to von Willebrand disease (vWD) type 2A, possibly as the large von Willebrand platelet coagulation factor (vWF) molecule suffers shear stress as it traverses the aortic valve.

The types of vWD are as follows:

I   heterozygous for gene defect, reduced levels of vWF
II   normal vWF levels but structurally abnormal
IIA abnormality in synthesis of vWF or with proteolysis
IIB increased function of vWF, leading to spontaneous platelet binding
III homozygous for gene defect resulting in severe bleeding tendencies

Edward Heyde, contemporary American physician

Erik Adolf von Willebrand, Finnish paediatrician (1870-1949)

10. Skin lesions (3)

B. Pemphigoid

Whilst we are not presented with a thorough history, and theoretically the man could have suffered multiple insect bites over the past few weeks, this would be extremely unusual, and even more so for the patient to not mention that he is living under constant assault. Stevens–Johnson syndrome and toxic epidermal necrolysis are both most often secondary to drug reactions, and we are not given a history of recent new medications started around the time of the start of disease. Stevens–Johnson syndrome is an extreme form of erythema multiforme (which gives classical "target lesions"), with bullae and systemic involvement including the pulmonary and renal systems, often with an extremely acute onset (rather than the subacute onset over weeks with which the man presented). Toxic epidermal necrolysis involves rapid widespread loss of large areas of the epidermis. Pemphigus does not present with such large, tense blisters, but rather with flaccid blisters and erosions in erythematous patches. These burst easily and heal very slowly. The Nikolsky sign, in which the skin of the blister can be made to slide off with the push of a finger, is characteristic in pemphigus. Oral involvement is very common. These are all in contrast to pemphigoid, which is far more common. They are both of autoimmune aetiology and the pathological difference is the site of the splitting – in pemphigus, the split is within the epidermis, whereas in pemphigoid the split is at the dermoepidermal junction. This is easily remembered as follows: pemphiguS = Superficial, pemphigoiD = Deep. Treatment of pemphigoid is with moderate doses of oral corticosteroids and often steroid-sparing immunosuppressants, such as azathioprine.

Pemphigus, from Greek *pemphix* = blister

Pyotr Nikolsky, Russian physician (1858-1940)

11. Antibiotics (2)

A. Ceftriaxone and tendon rupture

Tendon rupture has been reported rarely with quinolones such as ciprofloxacin. The risk is increased in elderly patients and when corticosteroids are used concurrently. Co-amoxiclav can cause a derangement in liver function tests with a cholestatic picture, occasionally leading to jaundice, but withdrawal of the antibiotic usually leads to resolution. Macrolides such as erythromycin increase gastrointestinal motility and thus commonly cause diarrhoea, however this has led to their intentional use as a prokinetic anti-emetic. Gentamicin can cause significant renal damage and hence the serum level of gentamicin is monitored during its use – increased levels suggest decreased urinary clearance due to nephrotoxicity and the interval between doses should be increased. Nitrofurantoin is no longer commonly used, only being indicated for uncomplicated UTIs, and pulmonary hypersensitivity reactions leading to fibrosis can occur.

12. Scoring systems (2)

E. Waterlow score

The Waterlow score is an important tool for assessing the risk of pressure sore development. Pressure sores are likely to develop in bedbound patients who have poor mobility, poor nutrition, incontinence and multiple co-morbidities. They can cause significant pain and become infected, leading to sepsis and even death. The Waterlow score is generally used by nurses during the admission of patients and is especially important in stroke victims, quadriplegics and comatose patients.

Waterlow J. Pressure sores: a risk assessment card. *Nursing Times* 1985

13. Investigation of headache (2)

D. Temporal artery biopsy

This woman has temporal arteritis. Giant cell arteritis (temporal arteritis) is an inflammatory vasculitis of the cranial branches arising from the aorta. It is commonest in the over 50s and is twice as frequent in females. Clinical features include general malaise, temporal headache, scalp tenderness and jaw claudication. Eventually, visual disturbance or visual loss can occur due to ischaemic optic neuritis caused by arteritis of the posterior ciliary artery and branches of the ophthalmic arteries. On examination, an enlarged, tender, non-pulsatile temporal artery is seen on the affected side. Temporal artery biopsy is the definitive investigation (shows patchy granulomatous inflammation) but skip lesions may be present and it is therefore possible that the histology is falsely negative. Investigation should not delay treatment with steroids. A CT and MRI of the head would not tell us much about the state of the temporal arteries or whether they are inflamed. The ESR is usually raised but this is non-specific. Ultrasound of the temporal arteries is relatively new and is being used as an adjunct to diagnosis.

14. Management of hyperglycaemia (1)

E. Start insulin infusion at 3 U/hour initially

This patient has developed a hyperosmolar non-ketotic coma (HONK). (See Paper 6 Question 47 Urinary frequency 2.)

15. Management of skin lesions (3)

A. Chemotherapy

This man has a basal cell carcinoma. The most common treatment for basal cell carcinoma is excision, as not only does this commonly remove all malignant cells, but it enables the diagnosis to be made histologically. It is most often done under local anaesthetic and complications are rare. In some circumstances other treatment modalities can be used. Mohs micrographic surgery aims for extremely narrow excision margins and histology is inspected at the time of excision to ensure the borders are clear, with repeat border trimmings until they are clear. This can be useful if there is limited local skin for closure or if there are nearby structures that are best avoided. Radiotherapy can be used to shrink lesions and reduce troublesome bleeding, often in cases where resection is difficult, either because of local invasion into certain structures or because the lesion is so large that flap reconstruction would be necessary and the patient is unsuitable for general anaesthetic. Topical 5-fluorouracil is commonly used for areas of skin with multiple or recurrent actinic keratoses, and can be used in some instances of basal cell carcinoma, although this is a relatively recent development. Chemotherapy has severe side effects and with such a range of effective local treatment options, and as basal cell carcinomas do not metastasise, chemotherapy is entirely excessive and not indicated.

16. Fatigue

E. Obstructive sleep apnoea

Obstructive sleep apnoea is characterised by episodes of complete or partial upper airway obstruction during sleep. Patients experience episodic airway obstruction associated with oxyhaemoglobin desaturation and arousals from sleep. The symptoms of obstructive sleep apnoea include chronic snoring, insomnia, gasping and breath holding, non-refreshing sleep and daytime somnolence. Maxillomandibular anomalies, adenotonsillar hypertrophy, an increase in soft palatal and tongue tissue mass due to obesity, and neuromuscular diseases with pharyngeal involvement leading to loss of dilator muscle tone cause narrowing of the upper airway during sleep. Treatment is by continuous positive airway pressure via a face mask during sleep.

17. Arterial blood gases (1)

B. pH 7.22, pO$_2$ 18, pCO$_2$ 2.3, HCO$_3^-$ 10

One of the consequences of acute renal failure is metabolic acidosis, and given that this man's renal failure was precipitated by sepsis, this is likely to be more marked as sepsis itself can cause metabolic acidosis. We are told that he was fluid resuscitated and treated with intravenous antibiotics, however, either the antibiotics have not been effective (and thus sepsis continues with vasodilation leading to renal hypoperfusion) or the fluid resuscitation has not been aggressive enough, or a combination of the two. His creatinine level has increased slightly and his urine output is very low at 8 ml/hour. His breathing, which is described in the scenario – deep and laboured in the absence of any respiratory problem (clear chest, normal saturations on air) – is called "Kussmaul breathing" and is a natural response to acidosis and aims to reduce the amount of acidic carbon dioxide in the circulation. As can be seen, the only acidotic blood gas reading with a low pCO$_2$ ("partial respiratory compensation") is option B. Note that the bicarbonate level is low, indicating a metabolic nature to the acidosis. Option A appears to be a respiratory acidosis with no metabolic compensation. Option C appears to be a mixed respiratory and metabolic acidosis with a high pO$_2$ – this may be due to oxygen therapy. Option D shows carbon dioxide retention with full metabolic compensation – this may be the blood gas reading of a patient with chronic obstructive pulmonary disorder. Option E is respiratory alkalosis with no metabolic compensation – this picture may be caused by a panic attack with hyperventilation in the absence of any bodily disturbance.

18. Shortness of breath (3)

B. Mesothelioma

Mesothelioma is a pleural tumour that is commonly associated with asbestos exposure. Shipyard workers, builders (mixing asbestos cement or fitting insulation), plumbers and electricians, who may be exposed to asbestos in their line of work, are more likely to develop asbestos-related lung disease. Breathlessness may be caused by a pleural effusion or circumferential pleural thickening. Computed tomography guided biopsy or thoracoscopy provides a definitive diagnosis. The prognosis of malignant mesothelioma is poor. The median survival in a variety of studies is between 8 and 14 months from diagnosis.

For more information, see the British Thoracic Society statement on malignant mesothelioma in the UK. *Thorax* 2007;62(Suppl2):ii1-19.

19. Management of chest pain

A. 24-hour ECG

This chest pain is probably cardiac in origin, secondary to paroxysmal tachycardia. This is best detected by 24-hour ECG. It lacks the correlation with effort of new-onset, stable angina secondary to coronary vascular disease. Any instance of tight chest pain or chest pain of sternal origin should be taken very seriously indeed. It is only because in this case she has not experienced the pain for at least 48 hours that a troponin blood test is not indicated – after this time it will not distinguish between a myocardial infarction (MI) and angina. An echocardiogram will detect valvular lesions and heart defects but it will not identify arrhythmias. Home oxygen is usually prescribed for patients with respiratory disease and chronic hypoxia after a full assessment; a cardiac patient so hypoxic that they need supplemental oxygen should not be sent home. Analysis of the 24-hour or ambulatory ECG will indicate the source of the tachycardia, i.e. supra-ventricular or ventricular (much more serious), which will in turn indicate a management plan that may include permanent pacing.

20. Barium enema

C. Crohn's disease

Barium enemas have largely been superseded by more advanced imaging and better endoscopy techniques but often still appear in exam questions. Described earlier are the signs of Crohn's disease. The main differential is ulcerative colitis, which would produce continuous changes from the rectum proximally and show a loss of haustra on plain film and a colon appearing shortened. The classical representation of colonic carcinoma is the stricturing "apple-core lesion". Coeliac disease is a condition involving the small bowel and so should not show signs on barium enema.

21. Cardiovascular examination

A. Dextrocardia

Inverted P-waves can be caused by dextrocardia or by the natural cardiac pacemaker being situated elsewhere in the atrium other than the sino-atrial node. In dextrocardia, the apex beat would be palpable on the right. The ECG leads should be reversed to yield a "normal" trace.

Dextrocardia is a congenital condition that may mean a normal heart is situated unusually rightward (dextrocardia of embryonic arrest and, as the name grimly suggests, is associated with malformations) or less commonly occurring as a mirror image on the right (dextrocardia *situs inversus*). If all internal organs are mirrored, it is known as dextrocardia *situs inversus totalis* (this is very rare). The latter two conditions are benign although they can occur in conjunction with primary ciliary dyskinesia (Kartagener syndrome).

Dextrocardia, from Latin *dextro* = right + Greek *cardia* = heart

Manes Kartagener, Polish physician (1897-1957)

22. Cauda equina syndrome

E. Upgoing plantars

The spinal cord ends with the conus medullaris around L2–L3, below which the dural sac simply contains the cauda equina, nerve roots that will exit at the lower lumbar and sacral spine. Saddle anaesthesia is due to compression of the sensory fibres leaving the spine at S3–S5. The bladder may be distended as detrusor motor paralysis and sensory loss leads to urinary retention. The lower motor neuron nature of the weakness reduces the anal tone, and may lead to reduced or absent ankle reflexes. The plantars would be expected to be downgoing, however. Plantars may be upgoing if there was compression higher up the spine, however there would not be the constellation of other signs mentioned here.

Cauda equina, from Latin *cauda* = tail + *equus* = horse

23. Joint swelling

C. Psoriatic arthropathy

In enteropathic arthritis, flares happen at the same time as flares of inflammatory bowel disease, and so given the absence of any such symptoms this diagnosis can be excluded. It also most commonly affects large joints of the lower limbs. Diffuse osteoarthritis affecting distal interphalangeal joints occurs far more frequently in postmenopausal females, and 35 years of age is very young for osteoarthritis. Psoriatic arthropathy has a typical onset between the ages of 25 and 40 years, and in 20% of patients it predates the appearance of psoriatic skin lesions (and in 5% there is never any skin involvement).

It is a diffuse disease category and there are five major patterns:

1. Distal interphalangeal joint predominance (seen here, most common in men, and most strongly associated with nail changes – onycholysis is the separation of the nail from the bed seen here, and pitting is also seen)
2. Asymmetrical oligoarthritis (commonly featuring dactylitis or "sausage fingers")

3. Symmetrical polyarthritis (resembling rheumatoid arthritis but less severe and not associated with nodules or other manifestations; it is more common in females)
4. Psoriatic spondylitis (less severe than ankylosing spondylitis)
5. Arthritis mutilans (also seen with rheumatoid arthritis; erosion of bone and cartilage in the fingers leads to telescoping).

Reactive arthritis is commonly found following dysentery or *Chlamydia* infection, and has a marked preponderance for lower limb involvement. It is associated with conjunctivitis in 50% of cases and also a non-specific urethritis (hence the mnemonic "Can't see, can't pee, can't bend a knee"). It is far more common in men than women (15:1). Enteropathic arthritis, psoriatic arthropathy, reactive arthritis and ankylosing spondylitis are the seronegative spondyloarthropathies and are heavily associated with HLA-B27, an immune histocompatibility gene (hence the relevance of the brother with Crohn's disease). Rheumatoid arthritis can be ruled out by the involvement of the distal interphalangeal joints.

24. Coeliac disease

B. Intestinal lymphoma

There is an eightyfold increased relative risk of intestinal lymphoma in coeliac disease compared to the normal population. These are predominantly T-cell derived lymphomas, and the risk is reduced with effective gluten exclusion. The other complications and associations listed are relevant to the inflammatory bowel diseases.

25. Complications of alcoholic liver disease

B. Delirium tremens

Delirium tremens is a syndrome of delirium, autonomic activation and agitation brought on by acute detoxification from alcohol. It is a terrifying and potentially life-threatening confusional state, with a 35% mortality rate if left untreated. It can progress to seizures and heart arrhythmias. In these patients it is important to monitor their vital signs as they can have precipitous drops in their blood pressure. Treatment is with benzodiazepines, such as chlordiazepoxide.

26. Diagnosis of abdominal pain (3)

A. Hypercalcaemia

Hypercalcaemia should always be suspected in patients with vague abdominal symptoms and known metastatic carcinoma, especially in malignancies prone to spread to the bone (breast, bronchus, kidney, prostate, thyroid and myeloma). Obviously in this scenario the most important differential to exclude is spinal cord compression. As well as malignancy, hypercalcaemia may be caused by primary hyperparathyroidism. Hypercalcaemia is said to cause "bones, groans, moans and stones", by this they mean changes to bone metabolism, abdominal pain, psychiatric symptoms and increased frequency of calcium stones. Treatment is initially supportive with good rehydration and identification and treatment of the underlying cause where possible. Bisphosphonates can also be used to lower serum calcium.

27. Disseminated intravascular coagulation

B. Increased fibrinogen

Meningococcal septicaemia can cause disseminated intravascular coagulation, as can a number of other infections (including *Escherichia coli*, *Streptococcus pneumoniae* and malaria) and other conditions including lung and pancreatic cancer. Diffuse endothelial damage leads to widespread tissue factor expression, thus activating intravascular coagulation and consuming platelets, factors V and VIII, and fibrinogen. Therefore the patient enters a haemorrhagic state. The INR and APTT both increase as both depend on factor V and fibrinogen. Platelets are used up in the coagulation and so fall, and haemoglobin is likely to fall with ongoing blood loss. However, the fibrinogen levels on the bloods should decrease as it is used in the intravascular coagulation. Treatment of the cause should be combined with platelets and/or fresh-frozen plasma as indicated by blood results and the clinical scenario.

28. Rectal bleeding

E. Urgent 2-week outpatient referral

In this scenario this bleeding may well be secondary to haemorrhoids, in that it is painless bleeding at the end of defecation. However, above the age of 60, any rectal bleeding warrants urgent investigation to rule out rectal carcinoma. Other criteria for urgent referral include a change of bowel habit for 6 weeks or more, unexplained iron deficiency anaemia and any palpable mass.

29. Diagnosis of cough (4)

C. Cystic fibrosis

Cystic fibrosis (CF) is the commonest autosomal recessive condition in the Caucasian populations in the UK, affecting one in 2500 live births. CF is caused by an abnormal gene coding for the cystic fibrosis transmembrane regulator protein (CFTR), located on chromosome 7. CFTR is a cAMP-dependent chloride channel blocker. The most common mutation in CF is the ΔF508 mutation. The poor transport of chloride ions and water across epithelial cells of the respiratory and pancreatic exocrine glands in CF results in an increased viscosity of secretions. The range of presentations is varied, including recurrent chest infections, failure to thrive due to malabsorption, and liver disease. In the neonatal period, infants may present with prolonged neonatal jaundice, bowel obstruction (meconium ileus) or rectal prolapse.

The gold standard investigation for CF is the sweat test. The abnormal function of sweat glands results in the excess concentration of sodium chloride (NaCl) in sweat. Sweat is stimulated by pilocarpine iontophoresis, collected on filter paper and analysed.

Normal sweat NaCl concentration = 10–14 mmol/L
Sweat NaCl concentration in CF = 80–125 mmol/L

At least two sweat tests should be performed, as diagnostic errors and false positives are common.

Management options in CF include physiotherapy (for respiratory secretions), antibiotics (for prophylaxis and treatment of lung infections) and pancreatic enzyme supplements (to prevent malabsorption). Complications include diabetes mellitus, hepatic cirrhosis, infertility in males, severe pulmonary hypertension and cor pulmonale, and chronic lung infections (*Pseudomonas aeruginosa* and *Burkholderia cepacia*). Many cases of CF are now being picked up early since the introduction of a national screening programme assessing immunoreactive trypsin (IRT) levels on the Guthrie card at day 8 of life. IRT is a pancreatic enzyme whose levels are raised in CF.

30. Diagnosis of gout

D. Crystals showing negative birefringence under polarised light

Calcium pyrophosphate crystals cause pseudogout. These are positively birefringent crystals and rhomboidal ("brick-shaped"). Apple green birefringence under polarised light is seen in tissues with amyloid deposits and stained with Congo Red. The negatively birefringent crystals of gout are spindle or needle shaped.

Gout occurs secondary to the deposition of uric acid crystals in the joint. It is commonest in older, obese male drinkers with hypertension, ischaemic heart disease and diabetes. Other risk factors include cytotoxic drugs, diuretic use and Lesch–Nyhan syndrome (gout + mental retardation + self-mutilating behaviour). Acute episodes of gout can be precipitated by trauma, illness, stress and thiazide diuretics. Acute gout usually presents with sudden pain, swelling and redness in the first metatarsophalangeal joint, although 25% of cases occur in the knee. Diagnosis is by joint aspiration, which shows negatively birefringent needle-shaped crystals. Acute gout is treated with non-steroidal anti-inflammatory drugs (NSAIDs, e.g. indomethacin, diclofenac). Prophylaxis is with allopurinol, a xanthine oxidase inhibitor that slows the production of uric acid. This is offered to patients who have recurrent gout, chronic gout, are using cytotoxic therapy, and those with Lesch–Nyhan syndrome. Allopurinol should not be prescribed within 1 month of an attack of gout as it may precipitate a further attack. In patients allergic to allopurinol, probenecid is used as prophylaxis.

Other forms of gout are chronic tophaceous gout (the accumulation of urate in cartilage, often the ear and Achilles tendon) and gout nephropathy (urate deposition in the kidneys resulting in acute renal failure and the formation of urate stones).

Gout, from Latin *gutta* = a drop. The ancient physician Galen thought that gout was caused by a small drop of the four humors in unbalanced proportions leaking into the joint space. The four humors - black bile, yellow bile, phlegm and blood - were thought to be the four basic substances of the human body, disturbances of which resulted in disease.

31. Investigation of shortness of breath (1)

C. Computed tomographic pulmonary angiography

Pulmonary embolism (PE) is a blood clot in the lung vasculature. Most PEs (75%) derive from a deep vein thrombosis. Features include acute-onset pleuritic chest pain and shortness of breath, often with fever and tachycardia. The chest X-ray may show a wedge-shaped opacity due to consolidation associated with pulmonary infarction (Hampton hump). The Westermark sign is a focus of oligaemia on X-ray distal to an occluded blood vessel. The ECG most commonly demonstrates a sinus tachycardia, although the S1Q3T3 pattern is characteristic (S-wave in lead I, Q-wave and inverted T-wave in lead III). An arterial blood gas reading reveals type 1 respiratory failure (normal pH, low pO_2). D-dimers are a breakdown product of clots: a low D-dimer can be used to exclude a PE, but a high level does not confirm it. The next investigation in PE depends on the chest X-ray: if the chest X-ray is clear, a ventilation–perfusion (V/Q) scan is performed to look for areas that are getting air but not blood. A normal ventilation–perfusion scan excludes pulmonary embolism in patients with low clinical probability, however a significant minority of high-probability scans are falsely positive. If the chest X-ray is not clear, or if a V/Q scan is inconclusive, a spiral CT (computed tomography pulmonary angiography (CTPA)) is the best investigation. Patients with good negative CTPA do not require further investigations and treatment for PE. It could also offer an alternative diagnosis when pulmonary embolism is excluded. Patients with a confirmed PE are started on heparin or low molecular-weight heparin and then warfarinised for 6 months (aiming for an international normalised ratio (INR) of between 2 and 3). Patients who have suffered a massive PE need urgent thrombolysis. Echocardiography is useful in diagnosis of massive PE. Acute dilatation of the right heart is usually present in massive PE with visible thrombus seen.

32. Diagnosis of neurological dysfunction (1)

D. Multiple sclerosis

Whilst she is concerned that this is Parkinson's disease, and there are some rare cases of early-onset familial Parkinson's disease caused by mutations in a single gene (for instance, alpha-synuclein, the misfolded protein that makes up Lewy bodies), not only is 27 still extremely young, but the clinical picture does not sound like Parkinson's disease. There is no sensory loss in Parkinson's disease, and the tremor is absent at rest and gets worse on movement (the opposite of the parkinsonian tremor). The tremor in fact sounds like an intention tremor. Regarding the symptoms being possibly psychogenic, this is common in young patients (especially female), however, there is no history of psychological abnormality, and the examination findings seem reliably reproducible and are consistent with certain anatomical lesions. Psychogenic neurology is often a diagnosis of exclusion after many investigations, although it is worth considering early on in certain patients who may start to deny the possibility of a non-organic cause.

The lack of an identified preceding infection does not preclude a postinfectious condition, either peripheral (Guillain–Barré) or central (acute disseminated encephalomyelitis – ADEM), and indeed the subacute onset could fit with such a diagnosis. With the leg symptoms, it is not known whether they are central (spinal cord) or peripheral. However, the intention tremor in the arm with lack of sensory symptoms or examination findings is most likely cerebellar in nature, and the cerebellum is not commonly affected in Guillain–Barré syndrome. Also, whilst Guillain–Barré syndrome can present initially with sensory symptoms, and it has only been 4 days since the start of the episode, weakness is usually a predominant feature and none was demonstrable on examination. This presents the possibility of ADEM or multiple sclerosis (MS). MS is the most common organic central nervous system disorder in the young, and affects women more than men, so this is the most likely. The feature in the history that supports this is the episode of visual blurring and eye pain (optic neuritis). ADEM is usually a monophasic condition, whereas MS, especially in the younger patients, commonly has a relapsing/remitting course with complete recovery in between relapses.

In the optic nerve, the axons conducting messages from the cone cells (colour vision and high acuity central vision) are myelinated, but those conducting messages from rod cells (dark vision and peripheral vision) are not, and so central vision and colour vision are more commonly affected.

The eye pain is commonly exacerbated on eye movement as the inflamed optic nerve sheath is stretched, however, this episode was mild and the hard-working patient has worked through it and forgotten such detail, so this is uncertain.

33. Management of multiple sclerosis

A. Baclofen

Baclofen is a gamma-amino-butyric acid (GABA)-derived drug commonly used as an antispasmodic. Oxybutinin is an anticholinergic used in detrusor instability and urinary continence issues in MS. MS sufferers can become constipated so lactulose (an osmotic laxative) can help. Modafinil is a stimulant drug sometimes used in MS to combat fatigue. Beta-blockers such as propranolol can help tremor.

34. Diagnosis of stroke

D. Right middle cerebral artery

The cranial nerve examination shows an upper motor neuron pattern of weakness on the same side as the limb weakness, and an homonymous hemianopia on the same side, which localises this stroke to the cerebral hemisphere rather than the brainstem. For that reason, the posterior cerebral artery cannot be the affected artery. The left-hand side of the body is affected, so it must be the right cerebral hemisphere – ruling out any artery on the left. That leaves us the right carotid, anterior cerebral or middle cerebral arteries. The arm and face being affected rules out the anterior cerebral, and the relative sparing of the leg (especially distal) indicates that it is the right middle cerebral artery territory that is affected. The right middle cerebral passes anterolaterally from the circle of Willis to lie on the outside of the hemisphere, before turning to run posteriorly in the Sylvian fissure, supplying the lateral part of all four lobes.

35. Diagnosis of cough (5)

B. Chronic obstructive pulmonary disease

This man has chronic obstructive pulmonary disease (COPD), as evidenced by a decreasing exercise tolerance and productive cough on a background of a smoking history. COPD is a chronic progressive disorder characterised by airflow obstruction. The obstruction may be partially (but not completely) reversible with bronchodilators. COPD encompasses bronchitis and emphysema. Chronic bronchitis is defined as cough with sputum for most days of a 3-month period on two consecutive years. Emphysema is a pathological diagnosis of permanent destructive enlargement of the alveoli.

Smoking is the main risk factor, and 15% of smokers develop COPD. The pathology includes hypertrophy of the goblet cells and decreased cilia with loss of alveoli elastic recoil. The persistent hypoxaemia seen in COPD results in pulmonary vascular hypertension, which leads to cor pulmonale. Features of COPD include a productive cough (worse in the mornings), recurrent respiratory tract infections, exertional dyspnoea, expiratory wheeze and bibasal crepitations. Examination may also reveal tracheal tug, intercostal in-drawing, a barrel chest (increased anterior–posterior diameter), pursed lips, central cyanosis, carbon dioxide retention (flapping tremor, bounding pulse and warm peripheries) and right heart failure.

COPD is diagnosed by demonstrating a forced expiratory volume in 1 second (FEV_1) of <80% and an FEV_1/VC (vital capacity) ratio of <70% with little variation in peak flow. The lung capacity and residual volume are increased. Arterial blood gases typically show hypoxia and hypercapnia. A chest X-ray shows hypertranslucent lung fields, a flat diaphragm, bullae and prominent hila. Management options include stopping smoking, antibiotics for infections, regular anticholinergics (ipratropium) and a salbutamol inhaler as required. Smoking cessation can be helped by bupropion, which is prescribed 2 weeks before stopping. Long-term oxygen therapy (LTOT) of 1–4 L/min via nasal cannulae is given for patients with severe COPD who have given up smoking and who have a pO_2<7.3 kPa and FEV_1 <1.5 L. Acute exacerbations of COPD are diagnosed when patients complain of worsening exercise tolerance, increasing sputum volume and increasing sputum purulence. Acute exacerbations of COPD are treated with 24–28% oxygen, nebulised salbutamol, oral prednisolone and prophylactic low-molecular-weight heparin. If CO_2 is rising or the patient is acidotic despite adequate oxygen therapy, consider ventilator support.

36. Management of diarrhoea

D. Oral vancomycin

The patient has become unwell as a result of the *C. difficile*-associated diarrhoea and needs treatment. Barrier nursing in a side room is recommended to limit spread of the organism, however it will not treat the patient. Co-amoxiclav and clarithromycin are not used to treat *C. difficile*, and in fact *C. difficile* associated diarrhoea often occurs secondary to antibiotic use disturbing the normal bowel flora. Omeprazole can also make infection more likely by reducing acidity of the bowel contents. Therefore, omeprazole and co-amoxiclav should be stopped, however this will not stop the infection now that it has started. The organism remains in the bowel lumen and causes diarrhoea by virtue of the toxin it produces, and intravenous vancomycin does not traverse the bowel wall and so oral vancomycin is the best treatment plan. Oral metronidazole is also effective and different hospital trusts differ in their policies.

37. Diagnosis of chest pain (3)

B. Gastro-oesophageal reflux disease

Differentiating gastro-oesophageal reflux disease (GORD) from a cardiac cause of pain can be extremely difficult. In this case the salient features are that the pain occurs on lying down to go to sleep. Although in unstable angina this may occur, you would also expect a patient to report pain on increased exertion as well. A GTN spray may relieve both GORD and angina as the nitrates cause smooth muscle relaxation in the oesophagus as well as coronary arteries.

GORD is associated with obesity, smoking, alcohol, hernias and pregnancy. Patients generally present with intermittent pain, or heartburn, which may be related to lifestyle factors such as large meals or alcohol. Medications can also contribute and should be reviewed. Endoscopy is not usually indicated for the diagnosis in young, otherwise healthy, patients, however urgent referrals should be considered in anyone over the age of 55 with new-onset symptoms or warning signs of weight loss, gastrointestinal (GI) bleeding or anaemia. Management of dyspepsia is by modification of lifestyle factors including weight loss, and pharmacological treatment with proton pump inhibitors. Complications of longstanding reflux are the development of Barrett's oesophagus and the formation of strictures.

38. Endocarditis

E. Two blood cultures positive for *Strep. viridans*, pyrexia of 38.5°C, splinter haemorrhages and Osler nodes, and new small cerebral abscesses

The Modified Duke criteria have two major criteria and seven minor criteria. To have a definite diagnosis of endocarditis, a patient needs two major criteria, one major and three minor criteria, or five minor criteria positive. A patient with one major and one minor, or three minor, may be said to have possible endocarditis.

The major criteria are:

- Blood culture findings (either typical organism from two cultures, positive blood cultures >12 hours apart, or three or more positive cultures taken over more than 1 hour)
- Endocardial involvement (either vegetations on echocardiogram or a new valvular regurgitation)

The minor criteria are:

- Predisposing cardiac/valvular abnormality (e.g. metal prosthetic valve)
- Intravenous drug use
- Pyrexia greater than or equal to 38°C

- Vasculitic phenomenon (e.g. petechiae, splinter haemorrhages, Osler nodes)
- Embolic phenomenon (e.g. cerebral abscesses)
- Blood cultures positive but not matching major criteria
- Echocardiographic findings suggestive but not matching major criteria

Comparing our patients, A has three minor criteria, B has one major criterion (the murmur sounds like mitral regurgitation) and one minor criterion (*Strep. viridans* accounts for 30–40% of endocarditis, but there is only one culture positive here), C has three minor criteria, D has one major criteria (blood cultures) and the murmur sounds like aortic stenosis that meets no criteria, and E has one major and three minor criteria. Diagnosis using the Modified Duke criteria is important to guide prognosis and management, which often involves a long regimen of multiple antibiotics (usually over 4–6 weeks).

Duke Endocarditis Service, Duke University Medical Center, Durham, NC, USA

39. Electrocardiogram (3)

C. Atrio-ventricular node re-entry tachycardia

Arrhythmias can be categorised as sinus node abnormalities, supraventricular or ventricular arrhythmias. Sinus bradycardia and sinus tachycardia are common sinus node abnormalities, and the P-waves remain associated with QRS complexes confirming normal functioning of cardiac conduction. The causes usually lie outside of the heart. Supraventricular arrhythmias include atrial ectopic beats, paroxysmal tachycardias (narrow complexes generated below the sino-atrial node but above the ventricles), Wolff–Parkinson–White syndrome (a separate pathway to the atrioventricular node (AVN) allows pre-excitation and re-entry), atrial flutter and atrial fibrillation. Atrial flutter is caused by a re-entry pathway allowing rapid re-firing of the ventricles: a rate of 300/min is typical. The AVN will often block some of the beats and additional P-waves appear at a regular rate of 300/min between QRS complexes. Atrial fibrillation is characterised by an irregular heart rate. Ventricular arrhythmias include ventricular ectopic beats, torsade de pointes, ventricular tachycardia and ventricular fibrillation. A broad QRS complex tachycardia indicates a ventricular arrhythmia (or a supraventricular arrhythmia with bundle branch block). AVN re-entry tachycardia occurs when two pathways co-exist within the AVN. The two pathways may have differing delays which in total, present a raised heart rate of between 140–220 bpm. These paroxysms can be managed with adenosine or verapamil to cause an iatrogenic AVN delay.

40. Ingested foreign body

D. Refer immediately to hospital for evaluation and possible endoscopic retrieval

Swallowing of foreign objects is a relatively common presentation in children. Most non-harmful objects can be managed expectantly and should pass through the gastrointestinal tract within 5–7 days. The parents should be asked to look for the object to ensure it passes. Anything that is potentially toxic, which includes batteries and sharp objects, or anything especially large, should be immediately referred to hospital for potential removal under endoscopy. The narrowest part of the GI tract is the oesophagus and this is the commonest site of impaction. If a battery becomes lodged in the oesophagus, removal is advised to avoid the small chance of oesophageal perforation. Once the object has passed into the stomach the chances of impaction are low.

41. Management of acne (2)

C. Oral lymecycline

Cyproterone acetate is an anti-androgen that may only be given to women, so it is contraindicated here. Topical steroid creams may be used when there are focal severe lesions, whereas this patient has diffuse but non-severe lesions. Oral prednisolone may only be used in severe cases, often where isotretinoin has not been fully effective. Systemic antibiotic therapy can be effective at clearing up acne, and often should be prescribed for over 6 months. Fat-soluble antibiotics are better delivered to the target (therefore penicillins are not preferred). Rather, tetracyclines or sometimes erythromycin are used.

42. Statistics (1)

C. 50%

The sensitivity of an investigation is its ability to detect a truly positive result. It is calculated as follows:

Sensitivity = number of true positives / (number of true positives + number of false negatives) × 100

In this case = 10 / (10 + 10) × 100 = 50%

43. Sexually transmitted infections (2)

C. Molluscum contagiosum

Molluscum contagiosum is caused by DNA-containing poxvirus. Spread is by sexual contact, personal contact and fomites (an inanimate object that is contaminated with disease-causing micro-organisms, such as a used towel). Hemispherical papules of 2–5 mm diameter that are pearly, raised and firm develop on the face, abdomen, buttocks and genitals. There is a latent period of 15–50 days. Spontaneous regression generally occurs, but lesions can be present for several months. Lesions can be extensive and persistent in immunocompromised patients, including those with HIV.

Molluscum, from Latin *molluscus* = a fungus (a particular type that grows on maple trees)

44. Management of shortness of breath (1)

B. Intercostal tube drain

Pneumothorax is the presence of air in the pleural space. It can occur spontaneously in healthy people (primary spontaneous pneumothorax) or in patients with pre-existing lung disease (secondary spontaneous pneumothorax). It can also result from iatrogenic injury or trauma to the lung or chest wall. Management of pneumothorax depends on the size of pneumothorax, clinical symptoms and underlying lung disease. The size of pneumothorax is divided into small or large depending on the size of the visible rim of air between the lung margin and the chest wall: <2 cm or ≥2 cm. Observation without any intervention is advised for small, closed, and mildly symptomatic primary spontaneous pneumothoraces and these patients do not require hospital admission. In patients with asymptomatic small secondary pneumothoraces, it is recommended to be admitted into hospital for observation. In patients with symptomatic primary or secondary pneumothoraces, active intervention is required as it may herald tension pneumothorax. Simple aspiration is recommended as first-line treatment for all primary pneumothoraces requiring intervention and mildly symptomatic small (<2 cm) secondary pneumothoraces. Intercostal tube drainage is recommended as first-line intervention in other symptomatic secondary pneumothoraces as they may cause respiratory failure. Tube drainage is also used if simple aspiration fails to control symptoms in any pneumothorax. Pleurodesis is to be considered to prevent recurrence in primary or secondary spontaneous pneumothorax.

45. Signs of liver disease (1)

B. Dupuytren contracture

Dupuytren contracture is a progressive fibroplasia of the palmar facia that results in a flexion contracture of the fingers. It is most common in the ring and little fingers. Risk factors include the male sex, a family history, diabetes mellitus, alcoholic cirrhosis, phenytoin use, trauma, acquired immunodeficiency disease syndrome (AIDS), Peyronie disease (idiopathic fibrosis of the corpus cavernosum) and Ledderhose disease (fibrosis of the plantar fascia, resulting in a similar deformity) On examination the thickened palmar aponeurosis can be felt. Treatment is by excision of the thickened part of the aponeurosis.

Trigger finger is characterised by difficulty in extension of a finger caused by a disparity in size between the flexor tendon sheath and the tendon within it. The finger remains flexed until passively extended with a "click". There is no association with alcohol excess.

Asterixis describes a jerking flexion–extension movement of the hand seen when the arms are placed in an outstretched position with the wrists cocked back. It is associated with hepatic encephalopathy and should be tested for in all patients with liver disease who present with an acute deterioration of disease, worsening ascites, confusion, agitation, reversal of sleeping pattern and stupor.

Guillaume Dupuytren, French surgeon (1777–1835)

46. Non-invasive ventilation

B. Home oxygen use

Non-invasive ventilation is now widely used in patients with chronic hypercapnic respiratory failure caused by chest wall deformity, neuromuscular disease or impaired central respiratory drive. It has a number of potential advantages, particularly the avoidance of tracheal intubation with its associated mortality and morbidity from problems such as pneumonia. According to the guidelines on non-invasive ventilation in chronic obstructive pulmonary disease (management of acute type 2 respiratory failure published by the British Thoracic Society) the inclusion criteria are: 1) primary diagnosis of chronic obstructive pulmonary disease (COPD) exacerbation (known diagnosis or history and examination consistent with diagnosis); 2) ability to protect airway; 3) patient is conscious and cooperative; 4) potential for recovery to quality of life acceptable to the patient; and 5) patient's wishes are considered. There is evidence to support the use of non-invasive ventilation in patients who are comatose secondary to COPD-induced hypercapnia in which endotracheal intubation is deemed inappropriate.

47. Systemic lupus erythematosus (1)

A. Anti-phospholipid antibodies

Anti-phospholipid antibodies (anticardiolipin or lupus anticoagulant) are present in 30% of SLE sufferers, and 2% of the population. The occurrence of repeated thrombotic events (arterial and venous) including miscarriages and transient ischaemic attacks (TIAs), as well as in cases of thrombosis at unusual sites, including cerebral or mesenteric circulations, should highlight the possibility of antiphospholipid syndrome. The first-line treatment is low-dose aspirin, but those with major thrombotic events such as a deep vein thrombosis (DVT) will often require anticoagulation with warfarin.

48. Medications in hyperkalaemia

E. Spironolactone

Amlodipine is a calcium channel blocker commonly used in hypertension and does not affect serum potassium. Bendroflumethiazide is a thiazide diuretic and actually lowers serum potassium. Whilst it is largely ineffective at lowering blood pressure in renal failure, it may be reducing the serum potassium and so shouldn't be stopped. Furosemide is a loop diuretic, which also lowers serum potassium. If this man has come in with acute renal failure caused by hypovolaemia, furosemide should probably be stopped. Simvastatin is a statin and does not affect serum potassium. Spironolactone is an aldosterone antagonist and will increase the serum potassium, and for this reason it should be stopped in renal failure, especially here, where the potassium level is raised. A serum potassium level of 5.5 mmol/L is not too high, but it should be checked that potassium is not being added to the patient's fluid prescription, as well as confirming that he is asymptomatic and checking his electrocardiogram (ECG) for changes.

49. Tumour markers

A. CA 125

The most likely diagnosis in this case is ovarian carcinoma for which CA 125 is a tumour marker. The clinical features of ovarian malignancy include weight loss, abdominal pain, increasing abdominal girth and ascites. Unfortunately, the symptoms of ovarian malignancy usually occur late, meaning the disease is often advanced and metastatic at presentation. Diagnosis usually involves transvaginal ultrasound scanning, computed tomography (CT) imaging, ovarian biopsy and measurement of CA 125. Both chemotherapy and surgery have a role in the management of ovarian cancer and have both curative and palliative roles. Radiotherapy is now limited to the palliation of symptoms. Because ovarian malignancy usually presents late the prognosis of ovarian cancer is poor. However, if the disease is diagnosed early and treated appropriately survival rates for early-stage disease can be as high as 95% at 5 years.

Other examples of tumour markers include:

Alpha-fetoprotein	$\rightarrow$	hepatocellular carcinoma, germ cell tumours

Beta-hCG	→	choriocarcinoma, testicular tumours
Ca 15-3	→	breast cancer
Ca 19-9	→	pancreatic cancer
Calcitonin	→	medullary thyroid cancer
Carcinoembryonic antigen	→	colorectal tumours
Monoclonal IgG (paraprotein)	→	multiple myeloma
Neurone-specific enolase	→	small cell lung cancer
Placental alkaline phosphatase	→	ovarian carcinoma, testicular tumours
Prostate-specific antigen	→	prostate cancer
S-100	→	malignant melanoma
Thyroglobulin	→	thyroid tumours

50. Parkinson's disease

D. Bradykinesia, postural instability, rigidity, and tremor ~3–4 Hz

Parkinson's disease symptoms are mainly caused by a lack of dopamine in the basal ganglia, secondary to a loss of midbrain substantia nigra pars compacta neurons. Models of basal ganglia function suggest that they take inputs concerning "motor plans" from the motor and cognitive frontal cortex, and then the dopamine acts as a gate to allow those motor plans to be executed. Hence, bradykinesia is a prominent symptom and is mostly related to the loss of dopamine. Postural instability appears late in the disease, and may be seen as a lack of ability to voluntarily adjust position in response to postural disturbance. Rigidity is classically either "lead-pipe" (stiff throughout range of movement) or "cogwheel" (essentially, lead-pipe rigidity with the tremor superimposed). The tremor of Parkinson's disease is the most common feature, and is usually unilateral and about 3–4 Hz in frequency. It may take the form of the classic "pill-rolling" tremor. A tremor of 10–12 Hz seems too fast for Parkinson's disease, and other causes such as familial or essential tremor should be considered. Postural hypotension may occur, but is more commonly a side effect of levodopa (L-DOPA) therapy, or associated with the "Parkinson-plus" syndrome, which is multiple system atrophy. Micrographia (small writing) and mask-like facies are features of Parkinson's disease but are less important diagnostically and functionally than the four main features.

James Parkinson, English surgeon (1755-1824)

Practice Paper 4: Questions

1. Airway management

You find an 80-year-old man collapsed in the street. He is unresponsive and is making a snoring sound. An ambulance has been called but has yet to arrive.

Which of the following is the best course of action?

A Cricothyroidotomy
B Do nothing till the ambulance arrives
C Finger sweep
D Head tilt chin lift
E Place in the recovery position

2. Management of pulmonary embolism

A 26-year-old woman presents to the emergency department with an oxygen saturation reading of 80% on air with a background history of increased breathlessness on exertion over the course of a week. She has not travelled abroad recently and does not have a family history of thromboembolism. On examination, there is elevation of the jugular venous pressure and accentuation of the pulmonary component of the second heart sound. A chest examination is unremarkable. A chest X-ray is normal and a subsequent CT angiography demonstrated a pulmonary embolism.

Which of the following management is NOT appropriate?

A Request an echocardiogram
B Request a thrombophilia screen
C Request tumour markers
D Start treatment dose low-molecular-weight heparin
E Start warfarin treatment

3. Skin manifestations of systemic disease (1)

A 34-year-old woman presents to the GP complaining of a new rash. The skin under her arms and on the back of her neck is dark and velvety in texture. She has a past medical history of diabetes for which she takes insulin.

What is the most likely diagnosis?

A Acanthosis nigricans
B Diabetic dermopathy
C Erythema ab igne
D Hyperhidrosis
E Xanthelasma

4. Scoring systems (3)

Which of the following scoring systems can be used to assess the risk of an adverse outcome following an upper gastrointestinal bleed?

A Breslow score
B CURB (Confusion, Urea, Respiratory rate, Blood pressure, Age) score
C Ranson's criteria
D Rockall score
E Waterlow score

5. Diagnosis of abdominal pain (4)

A 64-year-old man presents to the emergency department with a large rectal bleed and left-sided abdominal pain. He has a long history of constipation. He has a temperature of 38.4°C and a heart rate of 110 bpm.

What is the most likely cause?

A Angiodysplasia
B Bowel malignancy
C Diverticulitis
D Haemorrhoids
E Pseudomembranous colitis

6. Investigation of hepatomegaly

A 55-year-old man is being investigated for irregular heart rhythms. He has a medical history of diabetes mellitus. He explains that exercise is difficult for him due to joint pains. During the examination it is noted that he has tan skin pigmentation and hepatomegaly.

Which of the following investigations could reveal the aetiology of his symptoms?

A Haematinics
B Serum caeruloplasmin
C Short synacthen test
D Alpha-1 antitrypsin
E Gamma-GT

7. Substance use (1)

A 64-year-old woman is an inpatient on a surgical ward following an above-knee amputation. The nursing staff said she vomited earlier and she has been unresponsive since her operation a few hours ago. On examination, you noticed her pupils are small and she has a respiratory rate of 5 breaths/min.

Which of the following is the most likely reason for this clinical picture?

A Alcohol withdrawal
B Opiate use
C Opiate withdrawal
D Sedative use
E Sedative withdrawal

8. Home oxygen

A 66-year-old man with a 10-year history of chronic obstructive pulmonary disease is assessed in the respiratory clinic for eligibility for long-term domiciliary oxygen therapy.

Which of the following is NOT a criterion for prescription of long-term oxygen therapy?

A No exacerbation of chronic obstructive pulmonary disease (COPD) for the previous 5 weeks
B Patient has stopped smoking
C Patient has chronic hypoxaemia with PaO_2 <7.3 kPa
D Presence of pulmonary hypertension with PaO_2 <8.0 kPa
E Two arterial blood gases showing PaO_2 <7.3 kPa within 7 days

9. Management of chest pain (2)

A 68-year-old woman is recently not coping at home. She is now experiencing episodes of central, choking chest pain and shortness of breath on exertion. Her ECG is normal, as are her bloods and chest X-ray. Which of the following will NOT help her during her next episode?

A Bisoprolol
B Glyceryl trinitrate (GTN) spray
C Morphine
D Oxygen
E Salbutamol nebulisers

10. Antibiotics in pregnancy

A 33-year-old woman who is 10 weeks' pregnant develops increased frequency of urination and dysuria. Urine dip is positive for nitrites.

Which of the following antibiotics could be used to empirically treat the urinary tract infection?

A Ciprofloxacin
B Co-amoxiclav
C Doxycycline
D Trimethoprim
E Vancomycin

11. Left ventricular hypertrophy

An 80-year-old man attends the general practice for an annual check-up of his hypertension. He gingerly tells you all about his "left ventricular hyperthingummy". You check him and his records for confirmatory signs and symptoms.

Which of the following is NOT a sign of left ventricular hypertrophy?

A Inverted T-waves
B Left axis deviation
C Pansystolic murmur
D R-wave in V6 >25 mm
E The sum of the magnitude of the S-wave in V1 and R-wave in V5 >35mm

12. Shortness of breath (4)

A 79-year-old woman who was admitted to hospital with a fractured right neck of femur 1 week ago suddenly becomes acutely unwell on the ward 6 days after her operation. She complains of sudden-onset of shortness of breath and chest tightness. The pain is exacerbated by deep breathing. She has a past medical history of hypertension, hypercholesterolaemia and asthma. Her observations include temperature 37.8°C, pulse rate 108 bpm, blood pressure 96/66 mmHg, respiratory rate 26/min and saturations 89% on room air. On examination, her chest is clear to both auscultation and percussion. An electrocardiogram (ECG) shows sinus tachycardia without bundle branch block.

What is the most likely diagnosis?

A Acute exacerbation of asthma
B Myocardial infarction
C Pneumonia
D Pneumothorax
E Pulmonary embolism (PE)

13. Polycystic kidney disease (1)

A 43-year-old man presents with intermittent haematuria. On examination of the abdomen, bilateral masses are felt and an ultrasound reveals polycystic kidneys. You explain the syndrome to him. He is concerned that his son may develop the disease. He does not believe his wife suffers from the condition.

What is the probability that his son will develop the disease?

A Negligible
B One in two
C One in four
D One in a thousand
E One in two thousand

14. Management of status epilepticus

A 35-year-old homeless man presents to the emergency department unconscious and fitting. You estimate that he has been fitting now for 35 minutes. He smells of alcohol and looks dishevelled. He has an adequate airway and is breathing 10 L/min O_2. His pulse and blood pressure are within normal range, and his capillary glucose is normal.

What should your immediate management be?

A Diazepam 2 mg intravenously
B Diazepam 2 mg intravenously and Pabrinex intravenously
C Lorazepam 4 mg intravenously and Pabrinex intravenously
D Lorazepam 8 mg intravenously
E Lorazepam 8 mg intravenously and Pabrinex intravenously

15. Overdose and antidotes (2)

A 17-year-old female has taken 20 paracetamol tablets 3 hours ago in an attempt to end her life after an argument with her mum. She has now attended hospital with regret and is asking for treatment.

Which of the following should be administered?

A Atropine
B Desferrioxamine
C Digibind
D N-acetylcysteine
E Sodium bicarbonate

16. Murmur (2)

You are examining a tearful young child who has fractured her arm. On auscultation you hear an ejection systolic murmur. There is no cyanosis.

Which of the following prevents you reassuring her calm dad that his daughter has no serious heart problem?

A A history of cyanosis
B The fracture needs to heal first
C The second heart sound is split
D The murmur disappears on sitting up
E The murmur is soft

17. Management of shortness of breath (2)

A 60-year-old man presents to the emergency department with shortness of breath for 3 hours and chest pain. He also complains of a right calf pain that he has had for 2 weeks. He has a past medical history of hypertension, recent stroke and disseminated lung cancer. His observations include temperature 37.0°C, pulse rate 112 bpm, blood pressure 100/54 mmHg, respiratory rate 26/min and saturations 87% on room air. There is no significant finding on chest examination. An electrocardiogram (ECG) shows sinus tachycardia and new right bundle branch block. A computed tomography (CT) pulmonary angiography confirmed massive pulmonary embolism.

What is the most appropriate initial treatment?

A Intravenous caval filters
B Oral warfarin
C Prophylactic dose of low-molecular-weight heparin
D Thrombolysis
E Treatment dose of low-molecular-weight heparin

18. *Helicobacter pylori* infection

A 55-year-old man is found to have a gastric ulcer following an endoscopy for left upper quadrant pain. A rapid urease test is positive for *H. pylori* infection.

What treatment does this man need?

A H_2 antagonist plus metronidazole and clarithromycin
B Metronidazole, clarithromycin and amoxicillin
C PPI plus metronidazole and clarithromycin
D PPI plus H_2 antagonist plus an antibiotic
E Steroids + PPI + metronidazole

19. Management of hyperglycaemia (2)

A 55-year-old man presents to his GP with increasing lethargy and polyuria. He has a past medical history of ischaemic heart disease and congestive cardiac failure. He smokes 30 cigarettes per day and drinks alcohol occasionally. He has a body mass index (BMI) of 32. His random blood glucose is 14.0 mmol/L and fasting blood glucose level is 9.0 mmol/L.

Which of the following management is NOT appropriate in this patient?

A Advise the patient to change his diet and stop smoking
B Metformin should be considered as the first-line oral treatment option for overweight patients
C Sulphonylureas and metformin could be considered as a combined therapy if glycaemic control is not optimal
D Sulphonylureas should be considered if patient is intolerant to metformin
E Thiazolidinediones can be added to metformin and sulphonylurea combination therapy if control is not optimal

20. Drug administration

A 79-year-old woman is started on high-dose steroids for giant cell arteritis. As therapy will likely be maintained for at least a year, she needs bone protection. The decision is made to start alendronate 70 mg once weekly.

How would you advise her to take the tablet?

A Take it in bed at least half an hour before rising for breakfast
B Take it whilst sitting or standing just before breakfast
C Take it whilst sitting or standing upright at least half an hour after breakfast with minimal sips of water
D Take it with plenty of water whilst sitting or standing upright at least half an hour after breakfast
E Take it whilst sitting or standing upright at least half an hour before breakfast with plenty of water

21. Arterial blood gases (2)

A 59-year-old man is admitted to the emergency department following a fall. He complains of increased tiredness and jerking movement of his legs, which led to his fall from the staircase. He is a smoker. On arrival, he has an oxygen saturation level of 76% in air, and an arterial blood gas reading demonstrates: pH 7.40, PaO_2 6 kPa, $PaCO_2$ 9.3 kPa, HCO_3^- 35 mmol/L on room air. His respiratory rate was 20/min.

What does this blood gas result show?

A Acute type 1 respiratory failure
B Acute type 2 respiratory failure
C Compensated chronic type 2 respiratory failure
D Metabolic acidosis
E Respiratory alkalosis

22. Fluid therapy

A 55-year old man fractures his ankle attempting to replicate the latest dance fad he has seen his children do. He is otherwise fit and well and is haemodynamically stable. The fracture requires open reduction and internal fixation. The trauma registrar has said that he needs to be nil-by-mouth from midnight, however the operating list is always changing and new emergencies may come in. There are at least three cases that are likely to get done before him. Your request that he have breakfast as he is likely to be done later in the day is met with derision. He will need physiological fluid replacement when he is nil-by-mouth. He weighs 70 kg.

Which of the following regimens is closest to physiological needs?

A 1 L 0.9% normal saline with 20 mmol potassium and 2 × 1 L 5% dextrose in 24 hours
B 1 L 0.9% normal saline with 20 mmol potassium and 2 × 1 L 5% dextrose with 20 mmol potassium in 24 hours
C 2 × 1 L 0.9% normal saline with 20 mmol potassium and 1 L 5% dextrose in 24 hours
D 2 × 1 L 0.9% normal saline with 20 mmol potassium and 1 L 5% dextrose with 20 mmol potassium in 24 hours
E 3 L Hartmann's in 24 hours

23. Haemolytic anaemia

In haemolytic anaemia which is the correct pattern of investigations that you would expect to see?

A Low haemoglobin, low unconjugated bilirubin, high haptoglobin
B Low haemoglobin, high unconjugated bilirubin, high urinary urobilinogen, and low haptoglobin
C Microcytic anaemia, normal bilirubin, high transferrin, low ferritin
D Normocytic anaemia, normal bilirubin, low iron, low TIBC, normal ferritin
E Normal haemoglobin raised conjugated bilirubin, normal haptoglobin

24. Basic life support

You are the designated driver on Saturday night and are soberly walking to your car with your friends. You spot an elderly man lying on the ground. He is not breathing and has no pulse although he is warm. You ask a friend to call 999. His airway is clear. Your praecordial thump fails.

The most likely way for his heart to resume beating is:

A Adrenaline
B Defibrillation
C Cerebral reoxygenation
D Chest compressions
E Recovery position

25. Causes of tremor

Which of the following diseases is the most common reason for misdiagnosis of Parkinson's disease?

A Corticobasal degeneration
B Essential tremor/familial tremor
C Progressive supranuclear palsy
D Pugilist encephalopathy
E Wilson's disease

26. Biological therapies

A 46-year-old woman has been diagnosed with rheumatoid arthritis and has been on methotrexate for over a year, but sadly her disease is not under control. She wants to know about the new drugs used for rheumatoid arthritis that she heard about at a patients' association.

Which of the following statements about biological disease-modifying anti-rheumatic drugs (DMARDs) is NOT true?

A A chest X-ray should be taken before starting to rule out latent tuberculosis (which could be reactivated)
B If the patient's disease gets worse whilst on biological therapy, switching from one biological DMARD to another is unlikely to produce an improvement
C Injection site reactions for subcutaneously injected agents are common
D The more commonly used agents target and inhibit tumour necrosis factor alpha (TNF-alpha)
E They can be used in combination with methotrexate

27. Cognitive impairment (1)

A 55-year-old woman presents with mild cognitive impairment and disinhibition without significant mood change. She also has falls and urinary incontinence. She has no major past medical history or medications, and has never smoked or drank much alcohol. On examination, there are no cranial nerve or arm defects, however the legs appear to have increased tone, upgoing plantars and clonus bilaterally with some weakness of hip and knee flexion bilaterally.

Which of the following diagnoses may explain the picture?

A Alzheimer's disease
B Benign intracranial hypertension
C Lewy body dementia
D Normal pressure hydrocephalus (NPH)
E Vascular dementia

28. Complications of blood transfusion

A 45-year-old man is having his second transfusion following blood loss from a road traffic collision. During the transfusion he developed a fever of 38.5°C and rigors.

What should your immediate action be?

A Contact haematology for urgent advice
B Give steroids and antihistamines and continue transfusion
C Start antibiotics
D Stop the transfusion, take blood cultures and provide supportive measures
E Take blood cultures and continue transfusion

29. Diagnosis of numbness

A 32-year-old woman presents to her GP complaining of tingling and numbness around her mouth for 1 week. Occasionally, she also develops painful carpal spasm. She has a past medical history of Graves disease for which she just recently had subtotal thyroidectomy.

What is the most likely diagnosis?

A Hypercalcaemia
B Hypermagnesaemia
C Hypocalcaemia
D Hypophosphataemia
E Hypothyroidism

30. Diagnosis of postural hypotension

A 62-year-old woman presents to the emergency department with collapse. She felt dizzy when she tried to stand up from a sitting position. She did not lose consciousness. She denied any visual disturbances, headache or head injury. She also complained of fatigue over the past month. She takes only omeprazole and paracetamol. An ECG showed normal sinus rhythm. Blood pressure was 102/50 mmHg with a postural systolic drop of 30 mmHg. Blood test showed revealed Na^+ 126 mmol/L, K^+ 6.5 mmol/L, urea 10.0 mmol/L, creatinine 139 μmol/L.

Which of the following will be most useful in establishing the diagnosis?

A Low-dose dexamethasone suppression test
B Random cortisol level
C Renal ultrasound scan
D Short synacthen test
E Water deprivation test

31. Management of delirium

A 70-year-old man, admitted two days previously with a mechanical fall and needing rehabilitation, becomes increasingly anxious and agitated on the ward. He has been pestering the nurses for some "moonshine", and he is now disorientated in place and time. He claims to have seen little gnomes dashing between patients' beds. You suspect delirium tremens.

Which of the following represents best management?

A Intravenous Pabrinex
B Oral Pabrinex
C Reducing dose chlordiazepoxide
D Reducing dose chlordiazepoxide and intravenous Pabrinex
E Reducing dose chlordiazepoxide and oral Pabrinex

32. Liver function tests

Which of the below results is the best indicator of poor liver function?

A Raised alanine transferase
B Raised albumin
C Raised alkaline phosphatase
D Raised bilirubin
E Prolonged prothrombin time

33. Diagnosis of cough (6)

A 60-year-old woman presents to her GP with a chronic cough associated with thick, yellow sputum for the past year. Sometimes, the sputum is blood-tinged. She had been prescribed multiple courses of antibiotics but they did not seem to help. She had a past medical history of severe pneumonia that required admission to the intensive care unit for 20 days. On chest examination, there are inspiratory crackles throughout the lung fields, with normal vesicular breath sounds.

Which of the following is the most likely differential diagnosis?

A Bronchial carcinoma
B Bronchiectasis
C Chronic pulmonary obstructive disease
D Idiopathic pulmonary fibrosis
E Pneumonia

34. Diagnosis of skin lesions (1)

A 31-year-old man presents with a 1-month history of a growing round, flat, erythematous lesion on the left thigh. The border is slightly more erythematous than the rest of the lesion and has some flakiness of the skin. The lesion itches. The patient also has had long-standing itchy scales between his toes.

Which of the following investigations would help confirm the most likely diagnosis?

A Excisional biopsy
B Incisional biopsy
C Punch biopsy
D Skin scrapings to be sent for microscopy culture and sensitivities
E Skin swab to be sent for microscopy culture and sensitivities

35. Electrocardiogram (4)

A 56-year old man has a myocardial infarction the day after a hernia repair. You request an ECG and then compare it to his pre-admission trace. You notice ST-segment changes in leads II, III and aVF.

In which part of the myocardium is the infarct?

A Anterior
B Anterolateral
C Anteroseptal
D Inferior
E Posterior

36. Diagnosis of neurological dysfunction (2)

A 19-year-old female university student presents with problems in both arms and difficulty walking. Since starting her course she has had difficulty writing, typing, and other such activities, and thus has struggled to keep up with the workload. She says the arms have "felt unusual" for around 6 months. She describes finding small burns and blisters on her arms that she can't remember getting in the first place. In the last few weeks she has also fallen twice when walking up the stairs. The only other thing she describes is some mild occipital headaches that have increased in frequency lately. She is otherwise fit and well.

On examination, there is a loss of pinprick sensation found throughout the arms and on the back to around T3 level. Her hands appear to have some element of small muscle wasting and there is some loss of power throughout the arms. Reflexes are hard to elicit or possibly absent. In the legs, there is some mild symmetrical weakness, and the knee reflexes appear brisk. Plantars appear equivocal.

What is the most likely diagnosis?

A Cervical spondylosis
B Multiple sclerosis
C Psychogenic neurological symptoms
D Syringomyelia
E Viral transverse myelitis

37. Management of ischaemic stroke

A 74-year-old woman presents to hospital with an acute right-sided hemiparesis, and is found to have a left middle cerebral artery infarct on diffusion-weighted magnetic resonance imaging (MRI). It is her first stroke. Her past medical history is unremarkable. Her blood pressure is normal and her electrocardiogram (ECG) shows sinus rhythm with occasional ventricular ectopics. Blood tests show normal cholesterol and normal glucose. On carotid Doppler she is found to have an 85% stenosis of the left carotid.

Which of the following treatments will NOT benefit her?

A ACE-inhibitor
B Aspirin
C Left carotid endarterectomy
D Statin
E Warfarin

38. Malignant melanoma (1)

A 24-year-old woman who has been travelling to India on a gap year presents to clinic as she is concerned about a "funny-looking mole" on her leg. She is unsure how long it has been there.

Which of the following is not a concerning feature of a mole when considering a diagnosis of malignant melanoma?

A Asymmetry
B Bleeding
C Border irregularity
D Colour different to that of other moles on patient
E Itching

39. Nipple discharge

A 42-year-old woman presents to her GP with a 2-month history of nipple discharge from her left breast. The discharge is milky in colour. No blood is noted. She has a past medical history of hypertension, type 2 diabetes mellitus and depression. She has been taking regular medication for these conditions. She has been amenorrhoeic for 6 months. A provisional diagnosis of hyperprolactinaemia is made.

What of the following is NOT appropriate management?

A Breast examination
B Serum prolactin
C Stop antidepressants
D Thyroid function tests
E Urgent computed tomography (CT) of the brain

40. Palpitations (1)

A 52-year-old woman presents to the GP with intermittent palpitations and breathlessness that has occurred over the last few weeks. She denies chest pain. Her electrocardiogram (ECG) shows sinus tachycardia and she does not appear to be anaemic.

Which blood test would be of most use in confirming the diagnosis?

A Haematinics
B Lactate
C No blood test required
D Thyroid function tests
E Troponin

41. Diagnosis of endocrine disease

A 33-year-old man presents to his GP complaining of worsening headaches and tiredness for the last 2 months. He denies drinking alcohol and smokes occasionally. He has a good appetite and has gained 3 pounds over the past month. He also noticed that he has difficulty in biting his food, and has a reduced libido. On examination, he is tall, with an oval-shaped face, large hands and prominent lower jaw.

Which of the following tests is the most useful in the initial diagnosis?

A Growth hormone levels during an oral glucose tolerance test
B IGF-1 levels
C MRI scan of pituitary fossa
D Pituitary function test
E Random growth hormone levels

42. Emollient use

In which of the following circumstances would use of emollients be ill-advised?

A Acne vulgaris
B Contact dermatitis
C Eczema
D Psoriasis
E Wound healing

43. Medications in acute renal failure

An 83-year-old man is admitted with acute confusion. He has an extensive medical history including atrial fibrillation, type 2 diabetes, osteoarthritis, hypertension and some mild congestive cardiac failure, for which he takes several medications. He appears clinically dry, with a pulse of 115/min, dry mucous membranes and a capillary refill rate of 4 seconds. He is noted to have a reduced urine output with concentrated urine. His creatinine is 235 μmol/L.

Which of the following medications does not need be reduced or stopped?

A Amlodipine
B Diclofenac
C Digoxin
D Furosemide
E Metformin

44. Rectal bleeding (2)

A 27-year-old woman presents to the GP complaining of intense sharp pain on passing stools, accompanied by bright red bleeding noticed on the toilet paper. She has no fever and is otherwise well in herself. She recently had a course of codeine phosphate following a sprain injury to her ankle.

What is the most likely diagnosis?

A Anal abscess
B Anal carcinoma
C Anal fissure
D Crohn's disease
E Haemorrhoids

45. Signs of liver disease (2)

A 15-year-old girl is being investigated for behavioural changes and is found to have a green–yellow discolouration around her iris on slit lamp examination.

What is the name of this feature?

A Arcus senilis
B Caput medusae
C Kayser–Fleischer rings
D Lens dislocation
E Xanthoma

46. Indications for haemodialysis in acute renal failure

Which of the following is NOT an indication for haemodialysis in patients with acute renal failure?

A Acidosis with a pH <7.2
B Hypertension >220 mmHg systolic or 160 mmHg diastolic
C Persistent potassium of >7 mmol/L
D Refractory pulmonary oedema
E Uraemic pericarditis

47. Sexually transmitted infections (3)

A 43-year-old woman attends the GP with a 3-month history of a grey–white vaginal discharge which she says has a "fishy" odour. She is systemically well and has no menstrual abnormalities.

What is the most likely diagnosis?

A Bacterial vaginosis (BV)
B Candida
C Chlamydia
D Gonorrhoea
E Syphilis

48. Systemic lupus erythematosus (2)

A 35-year-old woman has had a diffuse mild arthralgia with a fluctuating time course for the last year. There is never much synovitis to be seen on examination and inflammatory markers are only mildly raised. ANA is positive.

Which of the following would make a diagnosis of systemic lupus erythematosus (SLE)?

A Anterior uveitis
B Anti-ribonucleoprotein antibodies
C Erosions on X-rays of affected joints
D Painful palpable purple lumps on the shins
E Red rash across the cheeks, worse in summer

49. Uraemia

Which of the following is NOT a sign of uraemia?

A Clouding of consciousness
B Hiccoughs
C Lemon yellow skin tone
D Spider naevi
E Twitching

50. Urinary frequency (1)

A 30-year-old man presents to the medical assessment unit with a history of excessive drinking and urination. He has been going to the toilet about 7–8 times per day for 1 month. His random blood glucose is 9.3 mmol. His results on admission show:

Na^+	130 mmol/L
K^+	3.5 mmol/L
Urea	2.4 mmol/L
Creatinine	80 μmol/L
Corrected Ca^{2+}	2.34 mmol/L
Plasma osmolality	609 mOsm/kg
Urine osmolality	145 mOsm/kg

Water deprivation test – urine osmolality 296 mOsm/kg after DDAVP 2 μg administered intramuscularly

What is the most likely diagnosis?

A Acute tubular necrosis
B Cranial diabetes insipidus
C Nephrogenic diabetes insipidus
D Primary polydipsia
E Type 2 diabetes mellitus

Practice Paper 4: Answers

1. Airway management

D. Head tilt chin lift

The head tilt and chin lift is the airway manoeuvre of choice when cervical spine trauma is not suspected. To achieve this, the patient is placed on their back and the rescuer simultaneously lifts the patient's chin whilst extending the patient's head. This simple manoeuvre lifts the collapsed soft tissues and restores airway patency. Once the manoeuvre has been completed the rescuer can reassess the airway by looking for chest movement and feeling for the patient's breath on their cheek. If the airway is patent and the patient is breathing spontaneously they can be placed in the recovery position. If the patient is not breathing, basic life support measures should commence.

2. Management of pulmonary embolism

C. Request tumour markers

Treatment dose of low-molecular-weight heparin and warfarin are standard therapy for patients with diagnosed pulmonary embolism. Thrombophilia screening should be considered in these patients with no known increased risk of venous thromboembolism. The examination findings suggest the presence of pulmonary hypertension and a transthoracic echocardiography could provide possible findings of right heart dilatation and a non-invasive assessment of pulmonary artery pressure.

3. Skin manifestations of systemic disease (1)

A. Acanthosis nigricans

The presence of a black, velvety overgrowth in the axillae, neck and groin is typical of acanthosis nigricans. This rash is associated with insulin resistance (diabetes), Cushing's syndrome, acromegaly, polycystic ovarian syndrome, lymphomas and adenocarcinomas of the gastrointestinal tract.

Other cutaneous features of internal malignancy include Paget's disease (scaly, eczematous rash on the nipple – breast cancer), thrombophlebitis migrans (recurrent thrombophlebitis in different parts of the body – pancreatic cancer), tylosis (hyperkeratosis of the palm and soles – oesophageal cancer), dermatomyositis (purple rash on eyelids and scaly pink rash on knuckles – lung and breast cancer) and necrolytic migratory erythema (blistering erythematous rash of buttocks, groin and legs – glucagonoma).

Diabetic dermopathy describes the presence of depressed pigmented scars in the shin. It is associated with diabetic microangiopathy. Other skin features of diabetes include necrobiosis lipoidica diabeticorum (shiny, atrophic yellowish–red plaques on the shins), cheiroarthropathy (a scleroderma-like thickening of the skin of the hands in insulin-dependent diabetics), granuloma annulare (small, papular lesions arranged in a ring and found on the back of the hands or feet) and acanthosis nigricans.

Erythema ab igne is a brown, lacy rash seen on skin that has been exposed to heat for long periods of time. It classically develops in hypothyroid patients who are cold and spend a lot of time in front of the fire. Excessive hot water bottle use can also result in the rash. Xanthelasma are yellowish plaques around the eyelid and may be due to hyperlipidaemia.

Acanthosis nigricans, from Latin *acanthosis* = thorn + *neger* = black

Ab igne, from Latin *ab* = from + *ignis* = fire

4. Scoring systems (3)

D. Rockall score

This scoring system can be used to predict adverse outcome following upper gastrointestinal bleeds by combining a number of independent risk factors (see below). A score of >8 indicates a 40% risk of mortality.

Factor	0	1	2	3
Age	<60	60–79	>80	
Shock	BP >100 mmHg, pulse <100	BP >100 mmHg, pulse >100	BP <100 mmHg	
Co-morbidities	None	IHD, cardiac failure	Renal/liver failure	Metastatic malignancy
Diagnosis	Mallory–Weiss tear	All other except malignancy	Upper gastrointestinal malignancy	
Endoscopy	None		Active bleeding, adherent clot, visible vessels	

Rockall *et al*. Risk assessment after acute upper gastrointestinal haemorrhage. *Gut* 1996; 38:316–321.

5. Diagnosis of abdominal pain (4)

C. Diverticulitis

A diverticulum is an outpouching of a hollow structure. Colonic diverticula are examples of false diverticula – the walls are made up only of the inner mucosal layer of the bowel. A true diverticulum involves all the layers of the wall from which it arises, e.g. Meckel diverticulum. Diverticulosis describes the presence of colonic diverticula. Diverticular disease is a term used if complications arise from diverticulosis. Finally, diverticulitis specifically describes inflammation of the diverticula.

Colonic diverticula are most commonly found in the sigmoid and the descending colon. They are unusual in the under 40s, but 30% of the elderly populations of developed countries are found to have diverticulosis at autopsy. The pathogenesis of diverticulosis is as follows: there is hypertrophy of the muscle of the sigmoid colon, resulting in high intraluminal pressures. This leads to herniation of the mucosa at potential sites of weakness in the bowel wall, which correspond to points of entry of blood vessels. The underlying aetiology of the initial large bowel hypertrophy is unknown, but it may be directly due to a diet that is chronically low in fibre. Complications of diverticulosis include diverticulitis, lower gastrointestinal haemorrhage from erosion of a blood vessel within a diverticulum, and obstruction from chronic diverticular infection and fibrosis. The diagnosis of diverticulosis is made by flexible sigmoidoscopy. Barium enema shows the diverticular outpouchings with a signet ring appearance due to filling defects produced by pellets of faeces within the diverticula. In the acute phase of suspected diverticulitis, computed tomography (CT) is the best investigation. Treatment of diverticulitis is largely conservative: patients are nil by mouth with the administration of intravenous fluids and antibiotics until symptoms improve. Complications of diverticulitis include the formation of abscesses (which may perforate, leading to peritonitis), fistulae and strictures.

Angiodysplasia can present with a similar picture, although there is less of an inflammatory response and bleeding is usually painless. There are small hamartomas within the gut wall that are liable to bleed. This is less common than diverticular disease but may be diagnosed on endoscopy.

Diverticulum, from Latin *di*= apart + *vertere* = to turn (i.e. a digression)

6. Investigation of hepatomegaly

A. Haematinics

The classical triad of haemochromatosis is bronze skin pigmentation, hepatomegaly and diabetes mellitus. Hereditary haemochromatosis is an autosomal recessive disease characterised by excess iron deposition in various organs throughout the body, which leads to their fibrosis and dysfunction. This question picks up on many of these complications: heart arrhythmias and possible heart failure; and skin pigmentation due to iron deposition in the hypothalamus leading to excess melanin production and hypogonadism. Iron deposition in the liver leads to acute liver failure, whereas deposition in the pancreas leads to failure of its endocrine or exocrine function. Joints are generally affected in an asymmetrical fashion. The diagnosis of haemochromatosis is made firstly from the haematinics, in which you would expect to see a raised ferritin, a reduced total iron binding capacity (due to saturation) and a transferrin saturation >60%. A liver biopsy will often show deposition of iron within the cells. The genetic loci for the common genes for haemochromatosis have also been located, with the two common mutations for the HFE gene being known. This can be useful in screening family members.

7. Substance use (1)

B. Opiate use

This patient is likely to be suffering the effects of opiate use. Examples of opiates include morphine, heroin, methadone and codeine. Effects of opiates (in addition to analgesia) include euphoria, nausea and vomiting, constipation, anorexia, hypotension, respiratory depression, tremor, pinpoint pupils and erectile dysfunction. The treatment of overdose (after AirwayBreathingCirculation (ABC)) is with the antidote naloxone. This is ideally given intravenously (but can be given intramuscularly or by inhalation). An infusion of naloxone may be necessary as the half-life is short. The effects of opiate withdrawal can be very extreme. They include dilated pupils, lacrimation, sweating, diarrhoea, insomnia, tachycardia, abdominal cramp-like pains, nausea and vomiting. Opiate dependence can be managed (once drug use has stopped) by methadone and buprenorphine (a partial agonist).

8. Home oxygen

E. Two arterial blood gases showing PaO$_2$ <7.3 kPa within 7 days

Long-term domiciliary oxygen therapy is the provision of oxygen therapy for continuous use at home for patients with chronic hypoxaemia of PaO$_2$ at or below 7.3 kPa (55 mmHg), nocturnal hypoventilation, and for palliative use. Long-term domiciliary oxygen therapy can be prescribed in patients with chronic hypoxaemia with a PaO$_2$ between 7.3 kPa and 8 kPa in the presence of pulmonary hypertension or secondary polycythaemia. The aim of therapy is to increase the PaO$_2$ to at least 8 kPa (60 mmHg) or to attain saturations of at least 90%. Studies have shown long-term domiciliary oxygen therapy used for ≥15 hours/day in patients with COPD and chronic severe hypoxaemia improves survival, reduces secondary polycythaemia and prevents progression of primary pulmonary hypertension. For patients who are eligible for long-term oxygen therapy, three factors should be considered:

1. There should be a clinical diagnosis of a disorder associated with chronic hypoxaemia.
2. Patients should be on optimum medical treatment for a particular condition and clinically stable for at least 5 weeks.
3. Arterial blood gas tensions must be measured on two occasions, not less than 3 weeks apart.

The patient should have stopped smoking and be made aware of the dangers of smoking in the presence of home oxygen therapy.

9. Management of chest pain (2)

E. Salbutamol nebulisers

This woman has stable angina. GTN spray sublingually causes peripheral vasodilatation, reducing afterload and resting her myocardium. Oxygen will ensure that what blood is perfusing her myocardium is well oxygenated, staving off hypoxia and its resultant anginal pain. Morphine is useful in calming the patient and reducing the unhelpful adrenal stimulus upon the heart. Bisoprolol is a beta-blocker that will serve to cap the heart rate by blocking the beta-adrenergic receptors. Salbutamol nebulisers are not only of no benefit in this scenario (the patient does not have restricted airways) but it also has functions as a beta-agonist, slightly stimulating the heart to work harder.

10. Antibiotics in pregnancy

B. Co-amoxiclav

Ciprofloxacin, a quinolone antibiotic, is contraindicated in pregnancy, as animal studies have shown development of arthropathy in the child. Tetracyclines, such as doxycycline, bind calcium and thus become deposited in growing bones and teeth, limiting growth and staining teeth. Trimethoprim is a folate antagonist and thus carries risk of teratogenicity. Vancomycin would have to be given intravenously, whereas this woman shows no indication of need for admission. This drug can cause severe side effects so is reserved for dangerous or resistant organisms, and it has only Gram-positive cover, whereas 75% of community-acquired urinary tract infections (UTIs) are caused by *Escherichia coli*, a Gram-negative organism. Co-amoxiclav provides good Gram-positive and -negative cover and is commonly used in UTIs. Penicillins are not known to be harmful in pregnancy.

11. Left ventricular hypertrophy

C. Pansystolic murmur

The heart can face an increased afterload in aortic stenosis, hypertension and raised peripheral vascular resistance. Its response, like any muscle, is to develop increased strength and therefore bulk. A larger muscle radiates a larger depolarisation charge, manifesting in an increased QRS amplitude and left axis deviation. This creates two problems: coronary arteries must traverse and support a thickened myocardium and end-diastolic volume is reduced as the larger myocardium intrudes upon the ventricular chamber. This can lead to acute coronary syndrome, signs of which include T-wave inversion. A pansystolic murmur can be a sign of mitral regurgitation, which is associated with left ventricular dilatation.

12. Shortness of breath (4)

E. Pulmonary embolism (PE)

Pulmonary embolism occurs in around 1% of all patients admitted to hospital and accounts for around 5% of in-hospital deaths. It usually arises from a venous thrombosis in the pelvis or legs. The clots break off and travel to the right side of heart via the venous system before lodging in the pulmonary circulation causing pulmonary circulation failure. The risk factors include any cause of immobility or hypercoagulability, e.g. recent surgery, pregnancy or postpartum, recent stroke or myocardial infarction, disseminated malignancy, thrombophilia and prolonged bed rest. A Wells' score is used to assess the clinical probability of a pulmonary embolism:

Clinically suspected deep vein thrombosis (DVT)	3.0 points
Tachycardia	1.5 points
Immobilisation/surgery last 4 weeks	1.5 points
History of DVT/PE	1.5 points
Haemoptysis	1.0 points
Malignancy (palliative or treated in last 6 months)	1.0 points
Alternative diagnosis less likely	−3 points

A score of <4 means a PE is unlikely, so consider measuring a D-dimer to rule out PE. A score of more than 4 means a PE is likely, so consider imaging (computed tomography (CT) pulmonary angiography).

Philip Wells, contemporary Professor of Medicine, University of Ottowa

13. Polycystic kidney disease (1)

B. One in two

The most common form of polycystic kidney disease has a prevalence of 1 in 1000 and is inherited in an autosomal dominant manner. Therefore, assuming that his wife does not suffer from the disease, the chance of his son being affected is 1 in 2. There is a rarer autosomal recessive form with a prevalence of 1 in 40 000.

14. Management of status epilepticus

C. Lorazepam 4 mg intravenously and Pabrinex intravenously

Diazepam or lorazepam can be used, but 2 mg of intravenous diazepam is too low a dose – 10 mg is the recommended dose. Lorazepam 4 mg should be used initially – then if there is no effect after 5 minutes, a further 4 mg can be used. Intravenous Pabrinex (vitamin B complex) is being used in this case as there is a possibility of alcohol withdrawal which, in the presence of B_1 deficiency (not unlikely in chronic alcoholism) can potentially cause Wernicke encephalopathy and then the irreversible Korsakoff syndrome – severe impairment of new memory formation, some impairment of accessing old memories, and confabulation.

15. Overdose and antidotes (2)

D. N-acetylcysteine

Paracetamol is widely available, cheap and extremely toxic in overdose. It is one of the most common drugs implicated in intentional overdose and is usually taken in combination with alcohol and other substances. There are usually no initial symptoms of paracetamol overdose, which often leads to the patient believing they have caused no harm. Late features of overdose include vomiting, abdominal pain, bruising, jaundice and encephalopathy. If a patient presents with paracetamol overdose, a serum paracetamol level should be tested 4 hours after the overdose was taken in addition to a full blood count, liver function tests, glucose and a coagulation screen. When a therapeutic dose of paracetamol is taken, the hepatotoxic metabolites are conjugated with glutathione, which neutralises their toxicity. In paracetamol overdose the endogenous glutathione pathways become saturated, allowing the hepatotoxic metabolites to build up and cause hepatic necrosis. N-acetylcysteine is the first-line antidote in paracetamol overdose and works by restoring the levels of glutathione, which conjugates and neutralises the toxins. It should ideally be started within 8 hours of the patient taking the overdose but can be given up to 24 hours after the overdose. If a patient presents more than 24 hours after overdose a specialist liver unit should be contacted for advice.

The decision to treat with N-acetylcysteine is usually based upon the serum paracetamol level taken at least 4 hours after the overdose. The paracetamol level is applied to a normogram that plots the time since overdose against the serum paracetamol level. On the normogram there is a low-risk treatment line and high-risk treatment line. If the patient's paracetamol level is plotted above the treatment line they will require N-acetylcysteine. If the patient is taking enzyme-inducing drugs or has pre-existing liver disease the "high-risk" treatment line should be used (which in practice means that this group are treated in the presence of lower serum paracetamol levels compared to patients who are not considered to be high risk). In cases of delayed presentation, extreme overdose, staggered overdose and unconsciousness it is often appropriate to treat prior to taking a 4-hour paracetamol level. If the patient has had a prior allergic reaction to N-acetylcysteine, the alternative antidote is methionine.

16. Murmur (2)

A. A history of cyanosis

Benign murmurs are common, especially in children. A Still murmur is a soft, ejection systolic murmur that disappears on sitting up (it is benign). Young children require vigorous cardiac output through comparatively narrow vessels; this can lead to a pulmonary flow murmur. The increased pulmonary vein pressure can lead to a delay in pulmonary valve closure – a split second heart sound. In children, the jugular vein walls can vibrate with the comparatively brisk venous circulation; this is known as a venous hum and is also benign. Fractured arms do not cause heart problems other than by secondary hypovolaemia – and dad would not be calm if this was the case! Ventricular septal defects are the commonest congenital cardiac defect and may present as a soft pansystolic murmur. If large, corrective surgery will be indicated; large defects ultimately cause cyanosis as an initial left-right shunt leads to an increased pulmonary vascular resistance reversing the shunt (and ending the cyanosis) – Eisenmenger syndrome. This will become a life-threatening problem and needs to be corrected.

Sir George Still also gave his name to juvenile idiopathic arthritis (Still disease) and was the first doctor to document attention deficit hyperactivity disorder in his lectures of 1902.

Murmur, from Sanskrit *marmara* = rustling sound

Victor Eisenmenger, Austrian physician (1864-1932)

George Frederic Still, English paediatrician (1868-1941)

17. Management of shortness of breath (2)

E. Treatment dose of low-molecular-weight heparin

If there is an acute massive pulmonary embolism that is accompanied by shock, thrombolytic therapy appears to improve outcome. However, in this case, the patient has high haemorrhagic risk and thus, it is not appropriate to administer thrombolytic therapy (e.g. alteplase). Anticoagulation therapy with low-molecular-weight heparin is effective in reducing mortality in pulmonary embolism by reducing the propagation of clot and the risk of further emboli. It is administered for at least 5 days and anticoagulation is commenced using oral warfarin.

18. *Helicobacter pylori* infection

C. PPI plus metronidazole and clarithromycin

Helicobacter pylori is a spiral-shaped Gram-negative bacteria found to be a causative organism in the development of gastric ulcers. It is able to colonise the harshly acidic environment of the stomach due to a urease enzyme that can locally convert urea into ammonia (which neutralises the surrounding acid) and carbon dioxide. *H. pylori* causes gastritis by inciting an inflammatory response from the host. It is implicated in gastric and duodenal ulcers as well as gastric carcinoma. There are several different tests available, including a C_{13} urea breath test, serological tests, tissue biopsy (rapid urease test, histology and culture) and stool test detecting antibodies to the bacterium. Eradication is via triple therapy (a proton pump inhibitor such as omeprazole, plus two relevant antibiotics) with a repeat endoscopy to show resolution of the ulcer.

19. Management of hyperglycaemia (2)

E. Thiazolidinediones can be added to metformin and sulphonylurea combination therapy if control is not optimal

Management of diabetes mellitus includes lifestyle changes and pharmacological treatment, including oral hypoglycaemics and insulin. Lifestyle changes such as regular exercise, having a healthy diet, and alcohol consumption reduction could improve glycaemic control. The aim of pharmacological treatment in diabetes mellitus is to lower the blood glucose level, which will provide relief from symptoms such as polyuria, polydipsia and reduce the risks of microvascular complications. Metformin acts by decreasing hepatic gluconeogenesis and improves peripheral glucose uptake while suppressing appetite and promoting weight reduction. It should be considered as the first-line oral treatment for patients with type 2 diabetes, especially when they are overweight. Sulphonylureas such as gliclazide and glipizide act by stimulating the release of insulin from pancreatic beta cells. They are considered in patients who do not tolerate metformin, or in those in whom it is contraindicated. Metformin and sulphonylurea could be considered as a combined therapy as they act synergistically. Thiazolidinediones work by activating peroxisome proliferator-activated receptor-γ, which regulates the expression of several genes involving metabolism, and work by enhancing the actions of endogenous insulin. They are used as a third-line therapy in combination with metformin and sulphonylurea, however they cause sodium and fluid retention and should not be used in patients with cardiac failure, such as in this case.

20. Drug administration

E. Take it whilst sitting or standing upright at least half an hour before breakfast with plenty of water

A dangerous side effect of alendronate is that it can cause oesophagitis, oesophageal erosions, oesophageal ulcers and oesophageal strictures. To avoid this, the exposure of alendronate to the oesophagus should be minimised. First, alendronate should be avoided in disorders that delay oesophageal emptying (e.g. strictures) and used cautiously in patients with dysphagia or reflux. Secondly, it should be taken upright so that gravity reduces transit time and reflux. Thirdly, by taking at least half an hour before any food, the chances of any alendronate refluxing into the oesophagus are reduced further. Fourthly, taking with lots of water should wash the alendronate through the oesophagus as swiftly as possible.

Owing to the complexity and inconvenience of taking alendronate, and frequent side effects ranging from dyspepsia to those mentioned earlier, there is often a poor compliance. If a patient on alendronate develops dysphagia or other oesophageal symptoms, it should be stopped. Intravenous bisphosphonates, which can be given less frequently (e.g. annual zoledronate) can be considered and are arguably more convenient but are more expensive.

21. Arterial blood gases (2)

C. Compensated chronic type 2 respiratory failure

A history of smoking suggests underlying chronic obstructive pulmonary disease. A $PaCO_2$ >6.0 kPa with a low pO_2 indicates type II respiratory failure, which would lead to respiratory acidosis. The pH can be expected to be acidotic, however in this case the pH is within the normal range and there is a high compensated bicarbonate level, which suggests chronicity, and compensated type 2 respiratory failure.

22. Fluid therapy

B. 1 L 0.9% normal saline with 20 mmol potassium and 2 × 1 L 5% dextrose with 20 mmol potassium in 24 hours

A man weighing 70 kg (average weight) requires 2.5–3 L of water a day, so all options are valid in volumatic terms. In terms of electrolytes, 140 mmol of sodium and 60–70 mmol of potassium are needed. A quantity of 1 L of normal saline contains 154 mmol of sodium. Hartmann's contains 131 mmol of sodium and 5 mmol of potassium, as well as chloride, calcium and lactate. As can be seen, 3 L of Hartmann's will give too much sodium and not enough potassium, which could lead to fluid retention and hypokalaemia, respectively. Therefore do not get caught by the "Hartmann's is more physiological" trap. Hartmann's may be more appropriate where there has been fluid and electrolyte loss (for instance, diarrhoea and vomiting). A quantity of 1 L of normal saline over the day will meet the patient's sodium needs, so it is between option A and B. Option A provides 20 mmol of potassium, and option B provides 60 mmol of potassium, therefore option B is the right answer.

23. Haemolytic anaemia

B. Low haemoglobin, high unconjugated bilirubin, high urinary urobilinogen, and low haptoglobin

Haemolytic anaemia is a pre-hepatic cause of jaundice. Haemolytic anaemia occurs when there is a shortening of the red cell lifespan, and biochemically this will present as an increase in the products of red cell destruction, as well as increased bone marrow cell production. There are many causes of haemolytic anaemia, either due to a cause within the red cell itself or within the vessel. Problems within the red cell can be with the membrane or with the production, such as sickle cell disease. Extrinsic causes can be divided into immune or non-immune causes. Haptoglobin binds free haemoglobin, therefore levels decrease where there is increased red cell breakdown.

24. Basic life support

B. Defibrillation

A praecordial thump upon the chest is only likely to cardiovert if given within seconds of a cardiac arrest. Chest compressions will move blood from the lungs to the cerebrum. This will prevent tissue hypoxia, leading to infarction and therefore reduce morbidity should the patient become successfully resuscitated, however they are unlikely to restore a pulse. Only defibrillation will start the heart beating again, although his airway should always be checked first as per the ABC protocol.

Praecordium, from Latin *prae* = in front of + *cordis* = heart

25. Causes of tremor

B. Essential tremor/familial tremor

The other four diseases actually cause genuine extrapyramidal symptoms and signs, however, essential/familial tremor is far more common. As tremor is the most widely known and usually the earliest sign of Parkinson's disease, and essential/familial tremor can present in late middle age, frequent misdiagnosis is understandable. Essential and familial tremor are similar, except essential tremor has no family history. These tremors are absent at rest but appear on action, have a frequency of 6–12 Hz and a fine amplitude, are present throughout the range of movement, and may be ameliorated by alcohol or beta-blockers. No other parkinsonian symptoms are present. The parkinsonian tremor is present at rest but diminishes with action, has a frequency of 3–7 Hz and a coarse amplitude, and commonly affects the distal limbs asymmetrically. Importantly, essential/familial tremor is separate from cerebellar tremor, which increases in magnitude throughout the movement to be maximal on approaching target, is usually 4–6 Hz, and is associated with other cerebellar signs.

Progressive supranuclear palsy combines parkinsonian symptoms with a supranuclear gaze palsy, most commonly and initially affecting downgaze. Wilson's disease is a disorder of copper metabolism leading to copper deposition throughout the body, most commonly in the liver (causing liver disease) and basal ganglia (causing parkinsonian and other extrapyramidal symptoms, e.g. dystonia), as well as the iris (Kayser–Fleischer rings). Usual onset is in the 20s to 30s. Pugilist encephalopathy is a parkinsonian syndrome resulting from repeated head trauma (a pugilist is a boxer). Corticobasal degeneration is an exceedingly rare syndrome with bradykinesia and an unstable posture with dystonias, alien limb phenomenon and apraxia (tremor is not a prominent feature).

26. Biological therapies

B. If the patient's disease gets worse whilst on biological therapy, switching from one biological DMARD to another is unlikely to produce an improvement

The relatively older biological DMARDs, which are less expensive (but still more expensive than traditional DMARDs) and have more long-term data and experience of use, target and block TNF-alpha, a key inflammatory cytokine. Etanercept is a humanised TNF-alpha receptor fused with IgG1, whereas adalimumab and infliximab are monoclonal antibodies to TNF-alpha. They can indeed reactivate latent tuberculosis and so a chest X-ray should always be taken before starting therapy to rule this out. Etanercept and adalimumab are given by subcutaneous injection (patients are taught to self-inject) and injection site reactions are a relatively common side effect. They work well alone but data suggests that they work better when used in combination with methotrexate. Other than the synergistic effect of using two DMARDs with different modes of action, it is thought that methotrexate may reduce formation of antibodies against the biological DMARDs themselves. Finally, switching between anti-TNF-alpha agents often can regain control of disease.

27. Cognitive impairment (1)

D. Normal pressure hydrocephalus (NPH)

Whilst falls and urinary incontinence can occur in Alzheimer's disease, these occur late in disease progression and do not fit with the patient's young age or mild cognitive impairment. Lewy body dementia has hallucinations as a prominent feature (which are not mentioned) and commonly coexists with parkinsonian movement symptoms. This woman seems to have pyramidal signs in the legs and no arm symptoms. Vascular dementia occurs with multiple strokes or transient ischaemic attacks (TIAs), which this woman does not have a history of, or risk factors for. Benign intracranial hypertension does not commonly cause dementia, and was mainly included to confuse, with its mention of intracranial pressure. It presents with headaches, visual disturbance (papilloedema, which would be absent with normal pressure) and sometimes VI cranial nerve palsies.

NPH commonly presents with the triad of dementia, gait disturbance and urinary incontinence. In NPH, cerebrospinal fluid (CSF) flow has been impeded but compensatory mechanisms have prevented raised pressure. The lateral ventricles are prominently dilated, and these ventricles exert local pressure on certain brain areas to give the classical clinical picture. Pressure on the frontal lobes gives the dementia and pressure on the medial side of the motor cortex, and the pyramidal tract fibres, cause incontinence and pyramidal leg weakness (remember the somatotopic organisation of the motor cortex in the precentral gyrus). Diagnosis is by lumbar puncture (to demonstrate a normal CSF opening pressure) followed by head computed tomography (CT)/magnetic resonance imaging (MRI) (showing enlarged ventricles). Treatment is with ventriculo-peritoneal shunting.

28. Complications of blood transfusion

D. Stop the transfusion, take blood cultures and provide supportive measures

Immediate transfusion reactions can be severe and potentially fatal. There are several possibilities for acute fevers during a transfusion. Rarely this may indicate an acute transfusion reaction, potentially due to ABO compatibility most commonly due to an error in administering the correct blood to the correct patient. This reaction will occur within the first few minutes of a transfusion and be characterised by shortness of breath, pain, and a fever (but the patient in this scenario is on his second unit). Very rarely a fever may be due to infection present in the blood product itself. A fever, especially following previous history of blood transfusion, may be due to a non-haemolytic transfusion reaction resulting from antibodies to the white blood cells.

In the acute setting initial management is vital to protect the patient. Initially this involves stopping the blood transfusion and providing supportive therapy to the patient, in terms of oxygen, hydration and ventilatory support as necessary. Senior help should be sought immediately, and the laboratory contacted to trace the blood to patient stocks. Steroids and antihistamines may be useful in calming the immune response in the short term. All transfusion-related adverse events must be reported to a centralised database that aims to improve overall safety.

29. Diagnosis of numbness

C. Hypocalcaemia

Hypoparathyroidism is a relatively common, and transient, complication of subtotal thyroidectomy. Reduced levels of parathyroid hormone result in high phosphate levels and low calcium levels. The symptoms of hypocalcaemia include perioral paraesthesia, muscular cramping and depression. Signs of hypocalcaemia include carpopedal spasm when a blood pressure cuff is inflated over the brachial artery (Trousseau's sign) and facial twitching when the facial nerve is excited by tapping above the parotid gland (Chvostek's sign). If the patient is stable and only suffering mild symptoms, the condition can be corrected using oral calcium supplementation. If the patient is very symptomatic, a 10 ml intravenous dose of 10% calcium gluconate can be administered. Approximately 1% of patients will develop permanent hypoparathyroidism following subtotal thyroidectomy.

The most common cause of hypocalcaemia is hypoalbuminaemia with a normal ionised calcium concentration (hence why it is important to correct calcium concentrations according to serum albumin). Other causes include alkalosis, vitamin D deficiency, chronic renal failure, pseudohypoparathyroidism, acute pancreatitis and hypomagnesaemia.

Pseudohypoparathyroidism is an autosomal dominant condition characterised by end-organ resistance to parathyroid hormone. Features include mental retardation, short stature and short fourth and fifth metacarpals, accompanied by a low PTH, low calcium and high phosphate levels. Pseudopseudohypoparathyroidism describes the condition where you get all the phenotypic features of pseudohypoparathyroidism but in conjunction with a normal biochemistry.

30. Diagnosis of postural hypotension

D. Short synacthen test

This patient presents with features suggestive of adrenocortical insufficiency, the diagnosis of which may be confirmed using the short synacthen test.

(For more information, see Paper 1 Answer 8 and Paper 2 Answer 26 on Collapse.)

31. Management of delirium

D. Reducing dose chlordiazepoxide and intravenous Pabrinex

Delirium tremens is caused by sudden alcohol withdrawal, and presents with agitation, confusion and hallucinations. Autonomic symptoms such as tachycardia, sweating, and nausea commonly co-exist. Lilliputian hallucinations (seeing little people) are characteristic. (Named after the island of Lilliput in Jonathan Swift's novel Gulliver's Travels, where the inhabitants were "not six inches high".) If untreated, seizures can occur. Chlordiazepoxide (a benzodiazepine) treats the agitation, and can prevent seizure occurrence, whilst B vitamin replacement aims to prevent Wernicke encephalopathy and the irreversible Korsakoff psychosis from developing (both caused by lack of vitamin B_1, levels of which can dramatically drop in alcohol withdrawal, especially with the likely malnourished state of the alcoholic). Pabrinex is not available orally, only intravenously. Chlordiazepoxide is commonly given as a high dose initially and then tailed off over 4–5 days.

Delirium, from Latin *delirare* = to be crazy (from *de* = away from + *lira* = path).

32. Liver function tests

E. Prolonged prothrombin time

The synthetic function of the liver is assessed either by the clotting pathway, as vitamin K dependent clotting factors are absorbed via the liver, or through serum albumin levels. If the liver is not functioning properly, clotting becomes deranged and the serum albumin concentrations decrease. Serum albumin, however, can act as an acute phase protein and be reduced in many inflammatory or infective situations. Alanine transferase and alkaline phosphatase are markers of hepatocellular damage.

33. Diagnosis of cough (6)

B. Bronchiectasis

Bronchiectasis is an abnormal permanent dilatation of bronchi secondary to destruction of the bronchial wall. It is usually an acquired condition as a consequence of recurrent and/or severe infections. It may result from an underlying genetic condition or congenital defect of airway defences. Patients present with a chronic cough that may be associated with large amounts of thick, yellow, foul-smelling sputum and sometimes haemoptysis. When there are large amounts of sputum in the bronchiectatic spaces, inspiratory squeaks and crackles and ronchi are heard on chest auscultation.

34. Diagnosis of skin lesions (1)

D. Skin scrapings to be sent for microscopy culture and sensitivities

This patient has tinea corporis in association with tinea pedis. Tinea is a fungal dermatophyte that can infect the skin in any area of the body. Common infections are tinea pedis (athlete's foot) and tinea cruris (fungal infection of the medial upper thighs). Tinea corporis is rarer and presents as a growing flat erythematous lesion with an inflamed scaly border. It usually spreads from tinea pedis on the same patient. Tinea pedis itself is usually transmitted by infected keratinous debris, e.g. from shower floors. Differentials of tinea corporis include granuloma annulare and erythema annulare. Fungal infection is confirmed by skin scrapings being examined under the microscope for fungal hyphae. Swabs are unlikely to pick up fungal material, and biopsies are excessive at this stage. If the skin scraping does not show a fungal element, and the lesion does not respond to empirical antifungal therapy, a punch biopsy may elucidate the cause and nature of the lesion and direct further therapy.

Tinea, from Latin *tinea* = growing worm

35. Electrocardiogram (4)

D. Inferior

Anterolateral infarcts typically show changes in V4–6, I and aVL. Anteroseptal infarcts show changes in V1–4. Anterior infarcts are shown in leads V1–6, I and aVL. Posterior infarcts rarely lead to substantial changes other than perhaps a raised R-wave in V1.

It helps to remember what the leads are measuring. II, III and aVF (F for feet) are measuring the downwards-pointing inferior myocardium. The chest leads and I measure the outwards pointing anterior myocardium (V1–4 right, V4–6 and I left). Infarcts usually occur in the harder working left ventricle, the right side of which is the interventricular septum.

36. Diagnosis of neurological dysfunction (2)

D. Syringomyelia

Let's start with the easy ones to rule out. Viral transverse myelitis is an acute illness and would not develop so insidiously. Cervical spondylosis is predominantly a disease that affects those over 50, and the arm signs would be more of a "radiculopathic" nature – shooting pains or paraesthesias in a nerve root distribution. This leaves two illnesses commonly presenting in young females: psychogenic symptoms and multiple sclerosis, and syringomyelia. Localising the potential lesion would identify the cervical spinal cord as the location (lower motor neuron signs in the arms, potentially upper motor neuron signs in the legs), so MS is a possibility. However, it does not sound like a normal relapse, as things have slowly progressed over 6 months with no clear resolution, and the symptoms and signs appear to be symmetrical. There is no evidence of brainstem, cerebellar or optic nerve involvement, and the white matter tracts appear to be less clearly involved than the lower motor neurons. Regarding the possibility of a psychogenic cause, the symptoms are not in a bizarre inexplicable distribution, and there are convincing examination signs, so that leaves syringomyelia.

In syringomyelia, the central canal of the spinal cord distends and begins to damage neurons by pressure effect. The syrinx (the swelling itself) starts in the cervical cord and can spread both superiorly and inferiorly. The first neurons to be damaged are the pain and temperature neurons bilaterally as their small axons cross the midline near the canal. As this only happens at the level of the syrinx and not above or below, and light touch and proprioception are spared, this causes the classic pattern of cape-like dissociated sensory loss. The anterior horn cell neurons (i.e. lower motor neurons) can also become damaged, giving a lower motor neuron picture at the level of the syrinx (wasting, absent reflexes), then long tract signs may develop later as the syrinx grows (upper motor neuron signs in the legs). Syringomyelia is usually associated with either a history of trauma to the spine, or the Chiari malformation, in which the cerebellar tonsils (at the very least) lie below the level of the foramen magnum. In this patient, she may well have the malformation, which may also explain the occipital headaches.

Syringomelia, from Latin *syrinx* = pipe or tube

Hans Chiari, Austrian pathologist (1851-1916)

37. Management of ischaemic stroke

E. Warfarin

Aspirin started immediately after an acute ischaemic stroke reduces early recurrence and has a small benefit on long-term outcome. Statin therapy has been shown to be beneficial even without high cholesterol prior to treatment. Warfarin is not indicated here as there is no atrial fibrillation, it is her first stroke and there is nothing sinister in the past medical history suggesting a drastic predisposition to thrombus formation. ACE-inhibitor therapy has a beneficial effect even if the blood pressure was previously normal. The European Carotid Surgery Trial showed that carotid stenosis

fossa is useful as hypersecretion of GH is normally from a pituitary tumour. Panhypopituitarism may also be caused by a pituitary tumour. IGF-1 concentration is high with excessive GH secretion, but in 25% of the cases, IGF-1 remains normal with increased GH secretion.

Acromegaly, from Greek acro = extremities + megalos = large

42. Emollient use

A. Acne vulgaris

Emollients, ranging from the thin aqueous cream to the far thicker "50:50" (white soft paraffin and liquid paraffin in 50% proportions) are useful in conditions featuring dry or scaly skin. They rehydrate the skin, reinstitute the surface lipid layer, and should be taken seriously as part of the management of dry or scaling conditions, without which other topical or systemic treatments would be less effective. Patient preference is a big factor and there is a wide range on the market, therefore patients should be offered many to find which ones suit them. Contact dermatitis, eczema and psoriasis would all generally benefit from use of emollients, by virtue of featuring dryness as part of the rashes. Emollients can also be applied to wounds during the healing process and this is encouraged by some surgeons. Acne vulgaris, however, is related to increased sebum production, which can block pores of sebaceous glands and become infected and inflamed. Therefore, emollients are only likely to make matters worse.

Emollient, from Latin emollire = to soften

43. Medications in acute renal failure

A. Amlodipine

Diclofenac is a non-steroidal anti-inflammatory drug (NSAID), which can be nephrotoxic by interfering with renal blood supply at the efferent arteriole, an effect magnified in hypovolaemia. Digoxin is excreted by the kidney and thus can have increased toxicity in renal impairment – the dose may need to be lowered. Furosemide is a potent diuretic and is likely to increase hypovolaemia and therefore should be stopped in this instance. Metformin can induce a metabolic acidosis and so should be stopped if the creatinine level is above 150. Amlodipine is a calcium-channel blocker, a relatively safe family of antihypertensives that does not need to be altered in renal failure, whereas angiotensin-converting enzyme (ACE)-inhibitors, beta-blockers and thiazide diuretics should all be used carefully in acute renal failure. If the patient becomes hypotensive, however, then it should be considered whether to stop the amlodipine for that reason.

44. Rectal bleeding (2)

C. Anal fissure

Anal fissures can occur in isolation, often following a period of constipation, or on a background of inflammatory bowel disease such as Crohn's disease. It is commonest in young people aged 20–30, and presents as an intense pain on defecation that may last for up to 1 hour afterwards. The pain is caused by a tear in the mucosa and muscle spasm during the passage of stools. Treatment is initially with stool softeners to attempt to allow the mucosa to heal naturally. Glyceryl trinitrite (GTN) topically may provide relief of symptoms, and botulinum toxin can be used where GTN fails.

45. Signs of liver disease (2)

C. Kayser–Fleischer rings

Kayser–Fleischer rings are seen in Wilson's disease, in which copper is deposited in vital organs due to an error in metabolism, which means that it cannot be secreted into the bile. Kayser–Fleischer rings are due to the deposition of copper in Descemet's membrane, which is located between the corneal stroma and endothelium in the eye. They appear as brown–green rings around the iris and are seen in up to 90% of patients with Wilson's disease. In most patients they can only be seen using a slit-lamp examination, although they may be visible with the naked eye in patients with light blue eyes and in patients with advanced disease.

46. Indications for haemodialysis in acute renal failure

B. Hypertension >220 mmHg systolic or 160 mmHg diastolic

Hypertension is not acutely life threatening, whereas acidosis, hyperkalaemia, pulmonary oedema and uraemic pericarditis can potentially be life threatening. Reliable pharmacological therapies that are not overcome by the ongoing renal failure exist for hypertension, whereas they do not for severe acidosis, persistent hyperkalaemia, refractory pulmonary oedema or uraemic pericarditis. Vasodilation and decreasing vascular resistance does not become impossible in renal failure. Acidosis can be temporarily ameliorated by use of sodium bicarbonate but it is unclear whether this helps in the long run, especially if the renal failure does not reverse. Severe hyperkalaemia can lead to ventricular fibrillation – monitoring should be instituted, calcium gluconate given to stabilise the cardiac membrane, and insulin with dextrose and calcium resonium given to lower serum potassium. However if the renal failure does not reverse, the potassium will continue to rise. Morphine can relieve respiratory distress and nitrates can vasodilate and pool blood away from the lungs in pulmonary oedema, but if the renal failure does not reverse, dialysis will be needed to remove the excess fluid. Acute rises in urea can lead to pericarditis and even pericardial effusions and tamponade, and only haemofiltration or haemodialysis can reduce the serum urea to prevent this if the kidneys do not soon recover.

47. Sexually transmitted infections (3)

A. Bacterial vaginosis (BV)

BV is not a sexually transmitted infection but rather an imbalance of the polymicrobial vaginal flora. There is often a preponderance of mixed anaerobic flora (e.g. *Gardnerella vaginalis* and *Mycoplasma hominis*). It is often asymptomatic, but can cause a creamy-grey discharge with a fishy odour. There is no itching. The diagnosis of BV is by the Amsel criteria (at least three of the following): homogenous discharge, clue cells on microscopy, pH of vaginal fluid >4.5, and release of a fishy odour on addition of 10% potassium hydroxide to the discharge. Clue cells are epithelial cells with bacteria adherent to the surface. BV can be treated with antibiotics (e.g. metronidazole) but there is a high rate of recurrence.

48. Systemic lupus erythematosus (2)

E. Red rash across the cheeks, worse in summer

Anterior uveitis often affects patients with ankylosing spondylitis or other HLA-B27-associated arthropathies. Anti-ribonucleoprotein antibodies can be involved in SLE but are more suggestive of the diagnosis of mixed connective tissue disease, which can give features of scleroderma, myositis and lupus. The arthropathy of SLE is normally non-erosive, and erosions are more suggestive of rheumatoid arthritis. Painful palpable purple lumps on the shins describes erythema nodosum, which may stand alone or be a feature of sarcoid, inflammatory bowel disease, or follow various infective diseases, e.g. post-streptococcal.

The red rash across the cheeks describes the classical malar or "butterfly" rash of SLE. Importantly, to make a diagnosis of SLE, the American College of Rheumatology criteria are used, and require four of 11 criteria to be fulfilled either serially or simultaneously (remembered by "A RASH POINts MD"):

- **A**rthralgia
- **R**enal disease → nephrotic syndrome
- **A**nti-nuclear antibody
- **S**erositis → pleurisy, pleural effusion, pericarditis
- **H**aematology disorders → pancytopenia
- **P**hotosensitivity
- **O**ral ulcers

- Immunology (autoantibodies) → anti-dsDNA, anti-Smith
- Neurological problems → depression, psychosis
- Malar rash
- Discoid rash

49. Uraemia

D. Spider naevi

Severe chronic uraemia can lead to a subtle pale yellow shade of skin that is described as "lemon yellow" or sometimes "uraemic frost". Uraemic encephalopathy can cause a clouding of consciousness and an acute confusional state, as well as myoclonic jerks, and this can progress to seizures and coma if not reversed. Hiccoughing is also seen. Spider naevi are seen in chronic liver disease and are not a feature of uraemia.

50. Urinary frequency (1)

B. Cranial diabetes insipidus

Antidiuretic hormone (ADH) is secreted from the posterior pituitary gland in response to a high plasma osmolality, hypovolaemia or stress. Its main function is to stimulate the reabsorption of water from the collecting ducts of the nephron into the circulation. This results in a reduction in plasma osmolality and urine output and an increase in urine osmolality and blood pressure. Diabetes insipidus (DI) is a condition caused by either an absolute lack of ADH secretion (cranial DI) or renal insensitivity to its actions (nephrogenic DI). DI usually presents with massive polyuria as water cannot be reabsorbed from the collecting ducts. As a result, patients with diabetes insipidus are often dehydrated and consume massive amounts of water in order to maintain their fluid balance. Other conditions that may present in a similar manner include diabetes mellitus, hypercalcaemia and psychogenic polydipsia. DI is suggested by a plasma osmolality of >300 mOsm/kg with a urine osmolality <600 mOsm/kg. Diabetes insipidus is usually diagnosed using the water deprivation test. This involves measuring the patient's urine volume, concentration and plasma osmolality whist depriving the patient of water. A positive result is recorded when water deprivation fails to increase the concentration of urine due to a lack of ADH or insensitivity to its actions. If the initial test is positive the patient is given a dose of desmopressin – a synthetic ADH analogue. If the patient concentrates their urine in response to desmopressin the defect must be central and a diagnosis of cranial diabetes insipidus can be made. If, however, the urine is not concentrated following desmopressin administration there is end-organ resistance to ADH, i.e. nephrogenic diabetes insipidus.

Diabetes insipidus, from Greek *diabainein* = to siphon + Latin *in* = not + *sapere* = to taste. In other words, to pass tasteless urine

Practice Paper 5: Questions

1. Alzheimer's disease

Which of the following statements regarding Alzheimer's disease is FALSE?

A Cholinesterase inhibitors may halt progression

B Computed tomography (CT) or magnetic resonance imaging (MRI) may show medial temporal atrophy

C Pathologically, extracellular beta-amyloid plaques are seen

D Pathologically, intracellular tau-protein neurofibrillary tangles are seen

E Short-term memory impairment is an early symptom

2. Antibiotics with warfarin

A 78-year-old man taking warfarin for a metallic aortic valve presents with 5 days of cough productive of purulent sputum, fever, anorexia and confusion. He is diagnosed with community-acquired pneumonia and is admitted for antibiotic therapy.

Which of the following antibiotics does NOT interact with warfarin?

A Ciprofloxacin

B Clarithromycin

C Gentamicin

D Metronidazole

E Rifampicin

3. Management of hyperglycaemia (3)

A 32-year-old man with known type I diabetes mellitus presents to the emergency department with nausea and vomiting. His blood glucose level was 24 mmol/L, with high blood ketones and K^+ 4.5 mmol/L.

Which of the following management is NOT appropriate in this patient on the first day?

A Commence intravenous 0.9% normal saline of 1 L over 1 hour

B Start intravenous insulin infusion at a rate of 6 U/hour

C Start intravenous K^+ supplement 40 mmol/L in the first bag of 0.9% normal saline

D Monitor blood glucose hourly

E Consider urinary catheter

4. Secondary prevention

Your consultant has heroically stented 72-year-old Mrs Harris' coronary arteries at 0200 hours over the weekend. Whilst reviewing her medication, she asks you what you think she could do to prevent this happening again and "spare these lovely nurses all this bother".

The best course of action would be to:

A Advise her that alcohol is not a cause of heart disease
B Ask her if she smokes and encourage her to cut down on salt intake
C Ask her if she smokes and review her long-term blood pressure and blood glucose
D Ask her if she smokes, check her lipid profile, review her long-term blood pressure and blood glucose and assess her pre-morbid mobility
E Encourage her to stop smoking and get out more

5. Investigation of hypothyroidism

A 43-year-old woman presents to her GP with a 3-month history of lethargy and low mood. She noticed that she had gained 2 stones over the past 2 months, despite having a normal appetite. On examination, she looked pale with periorbital puffiness, with a bitemporal hemianopia. Her thyroid gland was not palpable. Her thyroid function tests showed TSH 0.3 (range 0.5–5.5) mU/L , T4 3 (range 4.5–12.5) µg/dl.

Which investigation would be most useful in the diagnosis?

A 99m technetium (^{99m}Tc)scintigraphy scans
B Magnetic resonance imaging (MRI) of the brain
C Thyroid peroxidise antibodies
D Thyroid-stimulating hormone (TSH) receptor-blocking antibodies
E Ultrasound of the thyroid gland

6. Sickle cell disease

A 16-year-old boy with known sickle cell disease presents with painful hands bilaterally after being out early in the morning for a run. He is otherwise systemically well.

What should be your immediate management?

A Joint aspiration
B Malaria screen
C Referral to rheumatology
D Rehydration and analgesia
E X-rays

7. Substance use (2)

A 70-year-old woman has recently been admitted to hospital with a chest infection and mild confusion. Unfortunately no informant was available, hence a full history could not be taken. You are called to see her 2 days after her admission because she was sleeping poorly, complaining of nausea and sweating, and went on to have a seizure.

Which of the following is the most likely reason for this clinical picture?

A Alcohol withdrawal
B Opiate use
C Opiate withdrawal
D Sedative use
E Sedative withdrawal

8. Skin manifestations of systemic disease (2)

A 16-year-old girl presents to the GP with an itchy rash. This is located on both forearms and examination reveals evidence of blistering. She has a history of coeliac disease but is otherwise systemically well.

What is the most likely diagnosis?

A Acrodermatitis enteropathica
B Candidiasis
C Dermatitis herpetiformis
D Leukoplakia
E Linea nigra

9. Hepatic haemangioma

A 32-year-old woman undergoes a contrast enhanced CT scan of her abdomen to look for a cause of lower abdominal pain. Although no obvious cause of the pain is found, there is a small cavernous haemangioma of the liver.

What is the next step in management of this lesion?

A Anticoagulation with lifelong aspirin
B Chemotherapy
C Head CT to rule out cerebral haemangiomas
D No treatment necessary
E Surgical resection

10. Oxygen therapy

A 65-year-old man with a longstanding history of chronic obstructive pulmonary disease was admitted to the hospital with an acute exacerbation. His observations include temperature 37.5°C, pulse rate 120 bpm, blood pressure 140/90 mmHg, respiratory rate 28/min and saturations 84% on room air. An arterial blood gas shows pH 7.31, PaO_2 4.6 kPa, $PaCO_2$ 8.3 kPa and bicarbonate 25.2 mmol/L.

What is the most appropriate percentage of O_2 to be given initially?

A 28%
B 35%
C 40%
D 60%
E 100%

11. Polycystic kidney disease (2)

A 43-year-old man has just been diagnosed with polycystic kidney disease and is keen to know about potential risks or associated health problems.

Which of the following is not an extrarenal complication of polycystic kidney disease?

A Bladder diverticuli
B Cerebral aneurysms
C Hepatic cysts
D Mitral valve prolapse
E Pancreatic cysts

12. Myalgia

A 75-year-old woman presents with weight loss, anorexia and fatigue. She has lost 2 stone in weight in the last 6 months and she has been investigated for presumed dysphagia (she is not an excellent historian), which has found nothing. Her daughter said the first thing she noticed was a reduced walking ability and shoulder pain. You witness her struggle to stand up out of the chair. She also comments brushing the back of her hair is now difficult. She has tender shoulders to palpation. The blood tests reveal an erythrocyte sedimentation rate (ESR) of 60 mm/hour and a CRP of 30 mmol/L.

What is the most likely diagnosis?

A Fibromyalgia
B Inclusion body myositis
C Myasthenia gravis
D Polymyalgia rheumatica
E Polymyositis

13. Hyperbilirubinaemia

During a routine medical for a work placement a GP discovered that a 33-year-old man who was otherwise fit and healthy had a raised bilirubin level. He otherwise had entirely normal liver function tests and a full blood count. He had no history of foreign travel or drug or alcohol abuse. Repeated blood tests 1 month later showed a similar picture.

What is the most likely diagnosis?

A Crigler–Najjar syndrome
B Gilbert's disease
C Haemolytic anaemia
D Hepatitis B
E Pancreatic cancer

14. Drugs used in cardiac arrest

Which of the following drugs is used during cardiac arrest to improve the coronary perfusion pressure?

A Adrenaline
B Amioderone
C Atropine
D Calcium gluconate
E Magnesium sulphate

15. Management of thyrotoxicosis

A 35-year-old woman presents to the GP with increased weight loss over the past 2 months, with lid retraction, exophthalmos, and double vision. Her thyroid-stimulating hormone (TSH) receptor antibody level is raised.

Which of the following is the first-line treatment in this patient?

A Beta-blockers
B Carbimazole therapy
C Intravenous hydrocortisone
D Radioactive iodine therapy
E Subtotal thyroidectomy

16. Haemoptysis (1)

A 26-year-old woman from sub-Saharan Africa presents with two months of haemoptysis and lethargy. In the last month she has lost half a stone in weight and she frequently soaks the bedsheets with sweat. She has a negligible smoking history.

What is the most likely diagnosis?

A Lung cancer
B Lymphoma

C *Pneumocystis* pneumonia
D Pulmonary embolism
E Tuberculosis

17. Arterial blood gases (3)

A 33-year-old man presents to the emergency department with acute shortness of breath. He appears exhausted and unable to provide a clear history. An arterial blood gas reading shows pH 7.33, PaO_2 7.3 kPa, $PaCO_2$ 6.9 kPa and bicarbonate 26 mmol/L on room air.

What abnormality do these results represent?

A Metabolic acidosis
B Metabolic alkalosis
C Respiratory acidosis
D Respiratory alkalosis
E Type 1 respiratory failure

18. Dry eyes

A 38-year-old woman, with a history of autoimmune thyroid disease, presents with persistently dry eyes for over a year. She denies any arthralgia, rash, fatigue or any other symptoms. Schirmer's test reveals <10 mm wetting of filter paper in 5 minutes. Antibodies reveal positive anti-nuclear antibodies, with positive anti-Ro and anti-La antibodies.

Which of the following represents the best course of management?

A Artificial tears
B Hydroxychloroquine
C Steroids
D Surveillance
E Tear duct surgery

19. Management of shortness of breath (3)

A 21-year-old woman is admitted to the emergency department with increasing shortness of breath after taking oral amoxicillin, which was started by her GP for a chest infection. Chest auscultation reveals widespread wheeze bilaterally. Vascular access is secured.

Which of the following management options is NOT appropriate?

A Discontinue administration of the suspected drug
B Give intramuscular adrenaline immediately
C Give intravenous 5% dextrose immediately
D Give intravenous chlorphenamine
E Give intravenous hydrocortisone

20. Management of decreased consciousness

A 29-year-old man with known type 2 diabetes mellitus and excess alcohol intake was admitted to the emergency department with reduced consciousness. He is on oral anti-diabetic agents (intermediate and long-acting sulphonylureas) for his diabetes. His friend who brought him said that he had been drinking excessive quantities of alcohol that evening.

Which of the following managements is NOT appropriate in this case?

A Consider CT of the head
B Continue intravenous dextrose after the blood glucose level has returned to within normal range
C Intravenous dextrose
D Intramuscular glucagon
E Send random blood glucose sample to the laboratory

21. Haemophilia

Which clotting factor is deficient in haemophilia A?

A VII
B VIII
C IX
D XI
E vWF

22. Gastrointestinal pathology

A histology report for a specimen taken from the colon of a 24-year-old woman reports "patchy areas of transmural non-caseating granulomatous inflammation".

What disease process does this suggest?

A Colonic adenocarcinoma
B Crohn's disease
C Irritable bowel syndrome
D Tuberculosis
E Ulcerative colitis

23. Blood film

Which of the following conditions do not cause a leucoerythroblastic picture on blood film?

A Chronic myeloid leukaemia
B Megaloblastic anaemia
C Metastatic spread to the bone marrow
D Myeloma
E Tuberculosis

24. Lung cancer

A 55-year-old woman presents to the emergency department with a 1-month history of shortness of breath and weakness in both lower limbs. She has a 15 pack/year smoking history and has recently been diagnosed with diabetes by her GP. She has no other significant past medical history. On examination, there is reduced air entry on the left lower lung zone. Her chest X-ray shows a mass lesion on the left lower lobe.

An arterial blood gas reading shows: pH 7.53, PaO_2 8.6 kPa, $PaCO_2$ 5.3 kPa, bicarbonate 30.2 mmol/L.

The blood result shows: Na^+ 137mmol/L, K^+ 2.3, urea 4.8 mmol/L, creatinine 108 μmol/L.

A CT of the chest reveals a tumour invading the left lung and a percutaneous lung biopsy confirms the diagnosis of lung cancer.

What biochemical abnormalities are shown and what is the most likely histology of the lung cancer?

A Metabolic acidosis, non-small cell carcinoma
B Metabolic alkalosis, small cell carcinoma
C Metabolic alkalosis, non-small cell carcinoma
D Respiratory alkalosis, small cell carcinoma
E Respiratory alkalosis, non-small cell carcinoma

25. Cavernous sinus lesions

Which of the following cranial nerves would be affected by pathology in the cavernous sinus?

A II, III, IV and VI
B III and V
C III, IV and VI
D III, IV, VI and ophthalmic division of V
E III, IV, VI and V

26. Cognitive impairment (2)

A 75-year-old man presents with a history of episodes of cognitive impairment and memory deficits. His daughter seems perplexed that at some times he seems entirely normal, however some days he seems muddled and can't remember anything. He occasionally claims to see faces where there are none. He is a smoker and has chronic obstructive pulmonary disease (COPD), but there is nothing else in his past medical history. On examination he has a slow tremor present in his left thumb when relaxed or distracted, but not present when he is moving his arm. The arms appear to have a rigid tone, more on the left than the right. The rest of the neurological and general examination appears normal.

Which of the following is the most likely cause?

A Depressive pseudodementia
B Frontotemporal dementia
C Korsakoff psychosis
D Lewy body dementia
E Vascular dementia

27. Complications of bone marrow transplant

One year after bone marrow transplantation from a matched donor to treat non-Hodgkin's lymphoma a patient re-presents complaining of widespread skin irritation. The skin is exfoliated in areas and there is a maculopapular rash, while the fingers are becoming sclerotic. He has not been feeling himself for a while with episodes of diarrhoea and recurrent chest infections.

What is the most likely reason for this?

A Acute graft rejection
B Chronic graft-versus-host disease
C Herpes zoster infection
D New-onset scleroderma
E Side effect of immunosuppressants

Need More Help?

Go to the Athens page on our website

http://www.keele.ac.uk/healthlibrary/find/athens/

All NHS staff can apply for an Athens username. This will give you access to a wide range of subscribed online resources from any computer whether at home or work.

Salt
Sugar
Sex

HEALTH LIBRARY
North Staffordshire

Clinical Education Centre, University Hospital of North Staffordshire, Newcastle Road, Stoke-on-Trent, Staffs ST4 6QG

Tel: 01782 679500   Email: health.library@uhns.nhs.uk

A service for Keele University and the NHS in North Staffordshire

Web: www.keele.ac.uk/healthlibrary

28. Diagnosis of abdominal pain (5)

A 24-year-old woman presents with a 3-month history of vague right upper quadrant pains. She has also noticed an abnormal vaginal discharge since starting a new sexual relationship 4 months ago. On examination there is a hepatic friction rub.

What is the most likely diagnosis?

A Fitz-Hugh–Curtis syndrome
B Hepatitis C
C HIV
D Liver abscess
E Liver infarct

29. Diagnosis of cough (7)

A 36-year-old man has a 1-month history of a non-productive dry cough. He has also become more short of breath on exertion for the past 2 weeks. He was a known intravenous drug abuser. Chest auscultation is unremarkable. He is referred to the medical assessment unit for a chest X-ray, which shows bilateral symmetrical interstitial infiltrates. A subsequent HIV test is positive.

Which of the following is the most likely causative agent?

A *Aspergillus fumigates*
B Cytomegalovirus
C *Histoplasma capsulatum*
D *Pneumocystis jirovecii*
E *Staphyloccocus aureus*

30. Palpitations (2)

A 28-year-old woman with known neurofibromatosis type I presents to her GP with palpitations and recurrent headaches that are not relieved by paracetamol. She also feels dizzy and becomes sweaty during these episodes. Her blood pressure is found to be 220/120 mmHg.

What is the most likely diagnosis?

A Acromegaly
B Carcinoid syndrome
C Cushing's disease
D Thyrotoxicosis
E Phaeochromocytoma

31. Diagnosis of neurological dysfunction (3)

A 28-year-old Afro-Caribbean pregnant woman presents with a 2-month history of tingling in her feet and difficulty walking, which has progressed so that she is barely able to walk. She came to Britain 3 years ago from West Africa and has struggled to find work since, has a 2-year-old son, and lives in a flat with her boyfriend. She has been pregnant for 5 months. She has no significant past medical history other than various diarrhoeal illnesses when living in Africa – in particular she denies HIV. On examination, she looks thin and the conjunctiva are pale. There are no cranial nerve abnormalities, or abnormalities on the arms. In the legs, there is an increase in tone in the legs, with a marked weakness to about grade 3 or 4 throughout both legs, which is worse in the ankles. Knee jerks appear brisk, although the ankle jerks are hard to elicit and appear absent. Plantar reflexes are upgoing. There is a loss of light touch to just above the ankles, and there is absent proprioception and vibration sense in the big toe joints.

Which of the following is the most likely diagnosis?

A Diabetic polyneuropathy
B Guillain–Barré syndrome
C HIV-related polyneuropathy
D Subacute combined degeneration of the cord
E Tabes dorsalis

32. Diagnosis of skin lesions (2)

A 60-year-old man presents with a 1.5 cm raised pigmented lesion on his right arm. He is unsure how long it has been there.

Which feature on dermoscopy would suggest a malignant melanoma rather than a benign naevus or a pigmented seborrhoeic keratosis?

A Erythema of border
B Granular surface
C Irregular pigment network
D Stuck-on appearance
E Telangectasia

33. Malignant melanoma (2)

A 60-year-old Caucasian woman who recently moved from Zimbabwe presents with a growing pigmented lesion about 1 cm across with an irregular border and a raised, darker patch within. You suspect melanoma and excise the lesion.

Which of the following features of the tumour is the best prognosis indicator?

A Colour
B Diameter
C Grade

D Invasive depth

E Weight

34. Electrocardiogram (5)

Whilst on call, you are asked to review an ECG. It shows a long QT interval followed by a burst of QRS complexes at 300 bpm with an overlying waxing and waning R-wave amplitude, after which the ECG reverts back to its previous pattern. The patient feels well.

You conclude that this was an episode of torsade de pointes and should now:

A Advise the nurses to perform hourly observations

B Check the drug chart for possible causes

C Check the fluid balance chart

D Give anti-arrhythmics

E Send out a crash call

35. Diagnosis of chest infection (1)

A 75-year-old man presents with a 5-day history of cough productive of green sputum, mild right-sided chest pain, worsening breathlessness, and in the last day or so, confusion. He is previously fit and well with no background of dementia. He was in hospital 2 months ago for an elective hernia repair. On examination he has coarse crepitations at the right lung base, he has a respiratory rate of 34/min, a temperature of 38°C, and has an abbreviated mental test score of 6/10. Chest X-ray shows right lower zone consolidation and a small degree of blunting of the right costophrenic angle.

Which of the following is the likely diagnosis?

A Aspiration pneumonia

B Empyema

C Hospital acquired pneumonia

D Mild or moderate community-acquired pneumonia

E Severe community-acquired pneumonia

36. Emergency management (1)

A 16-year-old girl is seen by her general practitioner. She is lethargic and "not feeling her usual self" according to her parents. On examination, she has a stiff neck and a non-blanching purpuric rash on her trunk and legs.

Which of the following is the best course of action?

A Expectant management until there is deterioration

B Intramuscular benzylpenicillin and call ambulance

C Intramuscular benzylpenicillin and review in 12 hours

D Intravenous lorazepam and call ambulance

E Oral penciliin and review in 24 hours

37. Investigation of shortness of breath (2)

A 53-year-old retired truck driver presents to the general practitioner with a 3-month history of productive cough. He also complains of gradual onset of shortness of breath on exertion. He has to stop for breath after walking about 100 m on level ground. He is a heavy smoker, but is otherwise fit and well.

Which of the following investigations would be most useful in establishing the cause of his symptoms?

A Chest X-ray
B Electrocardiogram
C Peak flow meter
D Spirometry
E Sputum cytology

38. Diagnosis of chest pain (3)

A 54-year-old woman presents to her GP complaining of repeated incidents of burning central chest pain. It mainly occurs when she lies down to go to bed at night. She is overweight with a body mass index of 40. She uses GTN occasionally but it doesn't always relieve her symptoms. She doesn't report any shortness of breath or palpitations and examination is unremarkable.

What is the most likely diagnosis?

A Angina
B Gastro-oesophageal reflux disease
C Myocardial infarction
D Pancreatitis
E Sleep apnoea

39. Hypoxia

You are called to see a 92-year-old woman on the ward. The patient has been recovering from an exacerbation of heart failure. On arrival, the patient is on 15 L/min oxygen and an intravenous drip. You find the patient's oxygen saturation is reading 88% on pulse oximetry. She is having prolonged bouts of coughing, is reported by the sister as seeming physically weak for her, and is delirious.

Which of the following would be the most appropriate initial course of action?

A Check her fluid balance chart
B Check she is on regular paracetamol
C Keep checking the pulse oximeter hourly for deterioration
D Request a computed tomography (CT) pulmonary angiography
E Start her on antibiotics for hospital-acquired pneumonia

40. Management of hypothermia

A 46-year-old woman presents to the emergency department in a reduced state of consciousness. Her blood glucose level was 9 mmol/L. On examination, her body temperature was 33°C. She has non-pitting oedema on the skin of her hands, feet and eyelids. No obvious head injury is noticed. She has a thyroidectomy scar on her neck.

Bearing in mind the likely diagnosis, which of these is NOT appropriate in the initial management?

A High-flow oxygen if the patient is cyanosed
B Intravenous hydrocortisone
C Intravenous lorazepam
D Parenteral triiodothyronine, given slowly
E Warm blanket

41. Diagnosis of diabetes

A 45-year-old man presents to his GP with lethargy and polyuria for the past month. He has a strong family history of diabetes mellitus. A provisional diagnosis of diabetes mellitus is made.

Which of the following investigations is NOT useful in establishing the diagnosis?

A Fasting glucose level
B HbA1C level
C Oral glucose tolerance test
D Random glucose level
E Urine ketones

42. Medication review

An obese 48-year-old woman presented direct from work with fatigue and shortness of breath. She has been started on treatment for acute coronary syndrome but her oxygen saturation is now dropping and on review, you feel this is iatrogenic.

Which medication is most likely to be at fault?

A Aspirin
B Atenolol
C Clopidogrel
D Glyceryl trinitrate
E Heparin

43. Side effects of methotrexate

A 32-year-old woman is started on methotrexate for her newly diagnosed rheumatoid arthritis.

Which of the following is NOT true regarding side effects and contraindications of methotrexate?

A A baseline chest X-ray should be taken as pulmonary fibrosis is a potential side effect
B Alcohol should be absolutely avoided whilst taking methotrexate
C Full blood count should be monitored as neutropenia and myelosuppression are potential side effects
D Liver function tests should be monitored to watch for hepatic fibrosis
E Pregnancy should be avoided and if considering having a baby, methotrexate should be switched to an alternative disease-modifying anti-rheumatic drug

44. Raised intracranial pressure

A 55-year-old man presents to the hospital with a 4-month history of headaches, which usually occur in the mornings. These are becoming more frequent and severe.

Which of the following would suggest increased intracranial pressure?

A Jaw claudication
B Kernig's sign
C Low opening pressure on lumbar puncture
D Relief of symptoms when lying down
E Transient bilateral visual loss

45. Bronchial carcinoma

A 53-year-old man is seen in the medical assessment unit with lethargy, nausea, polyuria and polydipsia. He also has a weight loss of 2 stones over the period of 1 month. He smokes 40 cigarettes per day. A chest X-ray shows a lung mass in right lower lobe. His blood tests show a corrected calcium level of 3.1 mmol/L. Other causes of hypercalcaemia were excluded.

Which of the following cell types of bronchial carcinoma is most likely in this case?

A Adenocarcinoma
B Sarcomatoid carcinoma
C Small cell carcinoma
D Squamous cell carcinoma
E Large cell carcinoma

46. Neuro

A 44-y
histor
shoot
bad t
keyb
three
emin
thun

Whi

A (
B (
C I
D
E

47. [

int pain. She is concerned

OT used in the American
to diagnose rheumatoid
of arthritis?

ore than 6 weeks
more than 6 weeks
6 weeks

C Three or more j...

D Two hand joints (either metacarpophalangeal (MCP) or proximal interphalangeal (PIP)) involved for more than 6 weeks

E Ulnar deviation of one or more fingers for more than 6 weeks

48. Statistics (2)

A new tumour marker is being tested for use in cholangiocarcinomas. In a trial 40 patients have been tested. The trial produces 10 positive results and 30 negative results. Of the 10 positive results, 5 of them are false positives. Of the 30 negative results, 5 of them are false negatives.

What is the specificity of this test?

A 17%
B 50%
C 70%
D 83%
E 100%

Overlaid note:

Keep Your Athens Account Up-to-date

To edit your details or reset your password go to our Athens page and follow the instructions.

Logging in

To access our resources go to
http://www.keele.ac.uk/healthlibrary/find/healthinformationre sources/

http://www.keele.ac.uk/healthlibrary/find/athens/

This process is more efficient if you use an NHS network computer and an NHS-based email account.

nts with a 2-month
ess. The pains would
ought she was using
d despite ergonomic
She also says her first
wasting of the thenar
uced sensation in the
of her fourth finger.

49. Sepsis syndromes

A 43-year-old woman presents with a 1-week history of loin pain, suprapubic pain and dysuria. On examination she looks unwell, has a pulse of 110 bpm, blood pressure of 120/80 mmHg, respiratory rate of 24/min and a temperature of 38.5°C. Bloods are taken for routine tests and blood cultures, a catheter passed, and empirical antibiotics started. Later that day, blood cultures come back showing a Gram-negative rod. You note that in the last 3 hours she has only passed 30 ml of urine and she is starting to show signs of confusion. Observations remain as they were earlier.

Which of the following terms best describes the patient's physiological status?

A Sepsis
B Septic shock
C Septicaemia
D Severe sepsis
E Systemic inflammatory response syndrome

50. Nephrotic syndrome

A 38-year-old man presents with fatigue, swelling of the eyelids and legs, and frothy urine. His bloods appear normal except for an albumin level of 26 g/L (his albumin was normal on blood tests taken 1 year ago). You suspect nephrotic syndrome.

How would you confirm the diagnosis?

A Proteinuria on urine dipstick
B >1 g of protein lost in the urine over 24 hours
C >1 g of protein lost in the urine over 72 hours
D >3.5 g of protein lost in the urine over 24 hours
E >3.5 g of protein lost in the urine over 72 hours

Practice Paper 5: Answers

1. Alzheimer's disease

A. Cholinesterase inhibitors may halt progression

Short-term memory impairment is indeed an early symptom of Alzheimer's disease. The medial temporal lobe includes the hippocampus and other limbic system areas, and degeneration of these areas contributes to the impairment of memory function. CT or MRI may show this. On microscopic pathological examination of the brain, both extracellular beta-amyloid plaques and tau-protein-based neurofibrillary tangles are seen. Degeneration of the basal forebrain nuclei also occurs in Alzheimer's disease, and cholinesterase inhibitors increase functional acetylcholine at synapses, thus temporarily improving memory dysfunction, especially in early disease. Cholinesterase inhibitors, however, do little to halt the progression of the underlying neuronal loss and thus progression of disease.

Alois Alzheimer, German psychiatrist (1864-1915)

2. Antibiotics with warfarin

C. Gentamicin

Quinolones such as ciprofloxacin, macrolides such as clarithromycin, and the antibiotic metronidazole (used against anaerobic organisms) are all inhibitors of the cytochrome p450 metabolism system in the liver, and thus inhibit hepatic metabolism of the warfarin, leading to increased anticoagulant action and an increase in the international normalised ratio (INR). Rifampicin is a cytochrome p450 inducer, and so will enhance metabolism of warfarin and decrease the anticoagulant action. Aminoglycosides such as gentamicin are not known to affect the cytochrome p450 system. Not included as a potential answer here are any broad-spectrum penicillins such as amoxicillin. These do not affect the cytochrome p450 system, however, patients' INRs have been observed to rise when taking amoxicillin, and this is believed to be due to the effect on the gut flora. Many floral bacteria may break down warfarin before absorption, so the use of broad-spectrum antibiotics may lead to an effectively increased dose reaching the bloodstream.

3. Management of hyperglycaemia (3)

C. Start intravenous K⁺ supplement 40 mmol/L in the first bag of 0.9% normal saline

Diabetic ketoacidosis is a medical emergency that is characterised by the triad of cardinal biochemical features: hyperglycaemia, hyperketonaemia, and metabolic acidosis. A significant proportion of newly diagnosed type I diabetic patients present with ketoacidosis.

The hyperglycaemia causes dehydration and electrolyte loss, especially sodium and potassium through osmotic dieresis. Ketosis is caused by insulin deficiency, and it is exacerbated by elevated catecholamines and other stress hormones, resulting in unrestrained lipolysis to free fatty acids for ketogenesis in the liver. The resulting metabolic acidosis causes the exchange of hydrogen ions for intracellular potassium ions although there is also potassium loss through the kidney and intestine. Rehydration with intravenous fluids is essential but should be done with caution especially in the elderly. Insulin infusion is normally started at a rate of 6 U/hour in the first hour. The blood glucose level is monitored frequently for adequate adjustment of insulin therapy. A urinary catheter is considered in patients with oliguria for fluid balance monitoring. Potassium replacement is not needed in the first litre of intravenous fluid unless <3.0 mmol/L.

4. Secondary prevention

D. Ask her if she smokes, check her lipid profile, review her long-term blood pressure and blood glucose and assess her pre-morbid mobility

Smoking, high levels of low-density lipoprotein (LDL) cholesterol in the blood, hypertension, a lack of exercise and obesity are preventable risk factors for atherosclerosis and hence coronary artery disease. Poor management of diabetes and immoderate alcohol consumption cause hypertension and hence are secondary causes of atherosclerosis. The evidence that salt intake is as significant a cause of hypertension is not as conclusive. A doctor who engages with a patient rather than offering advice based on assumptions about them is more likely to achieve adherence.

5. Investigation of hypothyroidism

B. Magnetic resonance imaging (MRI) of the brain

Most cases of hypothyroidism in developed countries are caused by autoimmune thyroid disease and thyroid failure following ¹³¹I or surgical treatment of thyrotoxicosis. The symptoms are attributed to the infiltration of body tissues by the mucopolysaccharides, hyaluronic acid and chondroitin sulphate, resulting in a low-pitched voice and slurred speech due to a large tongue, and carpal tunnel syndrome due to compression of the median nerve. Non-pitting oedema is caused by the infiltration of the dermis, which is most marked in the skin of the hands, feet and eyelids. Hypothyroidism usually results from an intrinsic disorder of the thyroid gland, in which thyroid function test shows a low serum T_4 and elevated TSH level. In this case, however, the low serum T_4 and low TSH level suggest central hypothyroidism (secondary hypothyroidism), which warrants magnetic resonance imaging (MRI) of the brain to visualise a pituitary adenoma (which may explain the patient's bitemporal hemianopia).

6. Sickle cell disease

D. Rehydration and analgesia

A sickle cell crisis can involve several different pathological mechanisms, including vaso-occlusive, sequestration, haemolytic and aplastic. Crises are often precipitated by infection or dehydration. Homozygous Hb SS is associated with the most severe complications. In young males symptoms often appear during puberty, when there is a physiological rise in haemoglobin. The risk of a sickle cell crisis is avascular necrosis and joint deformity, which can occur in any bone or joint. The mainstay of treatment is analgesia, rehydration and oxygen therapy. Joints involved in sickle crises are prone to infection and therefore a low threshold is required before starting antibiotics.

7. Substance use (2)

E. Sedative withdrawal

This woman may be on long-term sedatives (benzodiazepines or barbiturates) that stopped being prescribed when she was admitted to hospital and was unable to give a clear medication history. Symptoms of sedative withdrawal include nausea and vomiting, autonomic hyperactivity, insomnia, delirium and seizures. Features of sedative use include loss of coordination, slurred speech, decreased attention and memory, disinhibition, aggression, meiosis, hypotension and respiratory depression.

8. Skin manifestations of systemic disease (2)

C. Dermatitis herpetiformis

Dermatitis herpetiformis is a blistering, intensely itchy rash that develops on the extensor surfaces. It is associated with coeliac disease and is treated with dapsone. Other cutaneous features of gastrointestinal disease include:

Malabsorption	→ Ichthyosis (dry, scaly skin), eczema, oedema
Liver disease	→ Jaundice, spider naevi, palmar erythema, leukonychia
Renal failure	→ Itching, half white and half red nails

Crohn's disease	→ Perianal abscess, fistulae, skin tags, aphthous ulcers
Ulcerative colitis	→ Erythema nodosum, pyoderma gangrenosum
Sarcoidosis	→ Erythema nodosum, lupus pernio (purple indurated lesions)

Acrodermatitis enteropathica is a rare inherited defect of zinc malabsorption. Features develop during weaning and include a perianal and oral red scaly pustular rash, failure to thrive, diarrhoea and poor wound healing. Oral hairy leukoplakia is a white rash that develops along the sides of the tongue that cannot be rubbed off (unlike *Candida*). It is caused by the Epstein–Barr virus infection and may be a sign of underlying human immunodeficiency virus (HIV) infection. Linea nigra is a dark line of pigmentation running down from the umbilicus that is a normal skin feature of pregnancy.

9. Hepatic haemangioma

D. No treatment necessary

Hepatic haemangiomas are common benign tumours of the liver present in 3–7% of the population. The majority do not cause any symptoms and are incidental findings. If a haemangioma is especially large or causing obstruction then it may be considered for surgical removal, otherwise no treatment is required.

10. Oxygen therapy

A. 28%

The ABG of this patient shows that he has type 2 respiratory failure with respiratory acidosis. The administration of high-flow oxygen will lead to worsening of the hypercapnic respiratory failure. In this situation, the oxygen therapy should be started at 28% or 24% using a venturi mask (controlled delivery) and modified depending on oxygen saturation and subsequent blood gas results. If oxygen administration results in failure of oxygenation or worsening hypercapnia, then non-invasive ventilation should be considered.

For further information, see the British Thoracic Society guidelines for emergency oxygen use in adult patients.

11. Polycystic kidney disease (2)

A. Bladder diverticuli

Cerebral aneurysms are associated with polycystic kidney disease, and thus the risk of subarachnoid haemorrhage is increased. For this reason, blood pressure should be monitored carefully and hypertension treated swiftly. Hepatic cysts and pancreatic cysts are associated, but only occasionally can be large and symptomatic (dull ache, acute pain caused by rupture, or obstructive symptoms such as obstructive jaundice). Mitral valve prolapse and mitral regurgitation are also linked. Bladder diverticuli are usually secondary to urinary outflow obstruction and can become infected due to stagnant urine or obstruction of their outlet. They are not associated with polycystic kidney disease.

12. Myalgia

D. Polymyalgia rheumatica

Polymyalgia rheumatica is a relatively common disease affecting 200 per million people above the age of 50 and largely affecting females from the age of about 70 upwards. Muscle stiffness and pain symmetrically affecting the proximal muscles is the classical presentation, but constitutional symptoms such as weight loss, fatigue and night sweats commonly occur. The ESR is typically raised above 40 mm/hour and this can be a clue to look for muscle stiffness, tenderness and weakness.

Fibromyalgia is a poorly understood disorder that has symptoms of widespread body pain and fatigue, but no associated inflammatory, structural, endocrine or metabolic abnormalities are found. It is associated with stress, poor sleep and altered pain processing. The presence of the marked unintentional weight loss would raise suspicion of an underlying pathological process, which is confirmed by the raised ESR and this rules out fibromyalgia.

Inclusion body myositis is a rare disease affecting mainly men over the age of 50 and more commonly involves the distal muscles (the fact that the affected person has difficulty standing and raising their arms suggests proximal muscle disease in the scenario), and there is no common large inflammatory component. Biopsy reveals rimmed vacuoles and inclusion bodies. It is not always responsive to steroids. Myasthenia gravis usually starts in the eyelids and muscles of the face before spreading to the body, and demonstrates the classical "fatiguing" phenomenon of weakness getting worse throughout the day and on repeated use of affected muscles (though this was not examined for in this scenario). Muscle tenderness is not usually an associated feature as the neuromuscular junction is the target of the autoantibodies rather than the muscle itself. Polymyositis is a rare (2–10 per million people) inflammatory myopathy that is sometimes paraneoplastic and normally affects those between 40 and 60 years of age. Weakness is often the main feature and pain and stiffness are not so prominent. The creatine kinase is often significantly raised.

13. Hyperbilirubinaemia

B. Gilbert's disease

Gilbert's disease (or Gilbert's syndrome) is a benign autosomal dominant partial deficiency in the glucuronyl transferase, the enzyme that's required to conjugate bilirubin. People with this condition have a mildly raised non-haemolytic unconjugated hyperbilirubinaemia, especially when they are acutely unwell. The remainder of the liver function tests are unaffected. Often this is picked up on routine screening, although some patients may experience intermittent jaundice. This condition requires no treatment.

Crigler–Najjar syndrome is a very rare autosomal recessive disorder of childhood caused by deficient metabolism of bilirubin. In this disease there is either a total or partial deficiency of hepatic glucuronyl transferase leading to high amounts of unconjugated bilirubin in the serum. Both types present with severe jaundice during the neonatal period and require phototherapy and phenobarbitone to reduce the levels of bilirubin in the serum. Although the milder form of the disease is treatable there is often some development of brain damage by adulthood.

John Fielding Crigler, American paediatrician (b. 1919)

Nicholas Augustin Gilbert, French physician (1858-1927)

Victor Assad Najjar, American paediatrician (b. 1914)

14. Drugs used in cardiac arrest

A. Adrenaline

Adrenaline interacts with alpha- and beta-adrenergic receptors to cause peripheral and splanchnic vasoconstriction, which divert blood away from the skin and gastrointestinal tract to the heart and brain. The net effect is an increase in coronary and cerebral perfusion pressures. Current resuscitation protocols advise that adrenaline is given as a 1 mg intravenous dose of 1:10 000 solution prior to the third shock and every 3–5 minutes thereafter in shockable arrhythmias (i.e. ventricular fibrillation and pulseless ventricular tachycardia). In non-shockable rhythms (e.g. asystole and pulseless electrical activity) adrenaline should be given at the start of the resuscitation attempt and every 3–5 minutes thereafter. Adrenaline is also available in a 1:1000 solution (where 1 mg = 1 ml). This solution should not be given intravenously and is reserved for use in anaphylaxis, when it is given intramuscularly.

Amiodarone is a membrane-stabilising drug that increases the refractory period of the cardiac cycle. Atropine is an anti-muscarinic drug that blocks the vagal nerve, thus increasing the rate of sinoatrial node and atrioventricular node depolarisation. Magnesium sulphate can be given as a 2 g (8 mmol) intravenous bolus in ventricular fibrillation refractory to defibrillation. Calcium gluconate stabilises the myocardium against the toxic actions of potassium, and is used in hyperkalaemia.

15. Management of thyrotoxicosis

B. Carbimazole therapy

The presence of eye signs and raised TSH antibodies suggests a diagnosis of Graves disease. Antithyroid drugs are used as first-line therapy in the management of Graves disease thyrotoxicosis. Antithyroid drugs such as carbimazole or propylthiouracil are given to the patient for a period of 12–18 months. These drugs reduce the synthesis of new thyroid hormones by inhibiting the iodination of tyrosine. Beta-blockers are used to control symptoms of thyrotoxicosis such as atrial fibrillation. If there is relapse, destructive therapy such as subtotal thyroidectomy or radioactive iodine therapy is recommended.

16. Haemoptysis (1)

E. Tuberculosis

Lung cancer can commonly cause haemoptysis but given the patient's age and smoking history this seems unlikely. Lymphoma can cause night sweats and non-specific malaise, and can present in patients of such an age, however the haemoptysis as a specific symptom must be looked into and lymphoma is not the most parsimonious diagnosis. *Pneumocystis carinii* pneumonia (PCP) can present with dry cough, fever and breathlessness in immunosuppressed patients. The haemoptysis and lack of breathlessness as a prominent feature go against the diagnosis. Pulmonary embolism can cause haemoptysis, however it would be acute in onset and typically feature chest pain and breathlessness. The insidious onset of haemoptysis with malaise and night sweats in a young person of sub-Saharan origin is highly suggestive of pulmonary tuberculosis. Multiple sputum cultures should be sent for Ziehl–Neelsen staining and culture, and a chest X-ray taken. Bronchoalveolar lavage can be performed if sputum is negative. Anyone presenting with tuberculosis should be counselled for HIV testing as it is far more common in immunosuppressed patients, and our patient's origin adds weight to this suspicion.

Tuberculosis, from Latin *tuberculum* = small lump (in reference to the primary lung focus)

17. Arterial blood gases (3)

C. Respiratory acidosis

Simple interpretation of arterial blood gases is usually all that is required in final SBAs. The pH value shows if the gas is acidotic (<7.35) or alkalotic (>7.45). Next, it must be determined whether the alkalosis or acidosis is due to a metabolic or respiratory cause – this is done by looking at the pCO_2 and bicarbonate levels. There are two things that must be borne in mind before continuing: 1) carbon dioxide is acidic and bicarbonate is alkaline; and 2) bicarbonate equates to "metabolic" and pCO_2 means "respiratory". Alkalosis can be due to either high bicarbonate ("metabolic alkalosis") or a low pCO_2 ("respiratory alkalosis"). Conversely, acidosis can be caused by either low bicarbonate ("metabolic acidosis") or a high pCO_2 ("respiratory acidosis").

In some cases of blood gas disturbance, the body has time to compensate. In other words, whichever chemical is causing the imbalance is counteracted by the opposite one. For example, if there is a high bicarbonate (metabolic alkalosis), then the pCO_2 starts to increase to raise the acidity and counteract the alkalosis. If compensation is successful, the pH will then return to within the normal range (7.35–7.45), even if the bicarbonate and pCO_2 levels are abnormal. It is important to know that the body can never overcompensate, i.e. if there is initial acidosis, the body can never make that into an alkalosis, and the pH will always remain on the acidic side of normal (pH <7.40). Similarly, compensated alkalosis will always have a pH >7.40, on the alkalotic side of normal.

Respiratory failure is defined as a pO_2<8.0. Type 1 respiratory failure occurs when there is hypoxia in the presence of a low or normal pCO_2. Type 2 respiratory failure is hypoxia in the presence of a high pCO_2.

In this case, the patient has type 2 respiratory failure (pO_2<8.0) with respiratory acidosis (low pH and high pCO_2).

18. Dry eyes

A. Artificial tears

At present her only symptom is persistently dry eyes, which is demonstrated by the positive Schirmer's test (see below). This is keratoconjunctivitis sicca, which in the absence of other rheumatological disease is primary Sjögren's syndrome.

The main features of Sjögren's syndrome are dry eyes (keratoconjunctivitis sicca) and dry mouth (xerostoma). Other features are corneal ulcers, oral candida, vaginal dryness, dyspareunia and respiratory hoarseness. Diagnosis is with Schirmer's test: a piece of filter paper 35 mm long is placed under the lower eyelid for 5 minutes – if less than 10 mm becomes moist it indicates

Sjögren's syndrome. Anti-Ro and Anti-La antibodies may be present. Treatment is with artificial tears and artificial saliva, as these help symptoms and carry little side effects. Surveillance therefore seems slightly cruel. Tear duct related interventions are rarely, if at all, indicated. Hydroxychloroquine can improve arthralgia and fatigue in connective tissue disorders, and steroids can be used in persistent salivary gland swelling or neuropathy (which can develop in association with Sjögren's syndrome), but neither are indicated here.

Henrik Sjögren, Swedish ophthalmologist (1899-1986)

19. Management of shortness of breath (3)

B. Give intramuscular adrenaline immediately

Anaphylaxis is a life-threatening condition caused by a severe allergic reaction to a certain allergen (e.g. drugs, food, insect stings, etc.). This leads to a systemic release of immune and inflammatory mediators from basophils and mast cells. It is normally initiated by an IgE-mediated hypersensitivity reaction. Patients present with bronchospasm and/or cardiovascular collapse. Patients should avoid further contact with the allergen. The airway should be maintained and oxygen should be provided at a high flow rate. Intramuscular adrenaline (0.5 ml of 1:1000 solution) is given immediately, followed by intravenous antihistamines. Corticosteroid is given to prevent late-phase symptoms, and has no role in the treatment of acute anaphylaxis. There is no evidence in using 5% dextrose for fluid resuscitation as it quickly redistributes itself out of the intravascular space. In the presence of associated hypotension, a colloid would be more appropriate.

20. Management of decreased consciousness

D. Intramuscular glucagon

Hypoglycaemia is defined as blood glucose <3.5 mmol/L. It is normally due to excessive amounts of insulin, either endogenous or exogenous. It commonly occurs in patients with diabetes mellitus using insulin, sulphonylureas or rarely metformin. Common symptoms of hypoglycaemia include sweating, anxiety, tremor, or in severe hypoglycaemia speech difficulty, confusion and reduced consciousness. When glucose values drop below the normal fasting range, the glucose meters are not accurate and a laboratory specimen is needed to confirm hypoglycaemia. Oral glucose drinks can be given to those who are conscious and able to swallow, while intravenous dextrose is given to those who have impaired consciousness or in severe hypoglycaemia. In patients on intermediate or long-acting insulin or long-acting sulphonylureas, there is a possibility of recurrent hypoglycaemia and they should be given intravenous dextrose titrated to blood glucose to prevent recurrence. Given the strong history of alcoholism, a CT of the head should be considered in this case as alcoholism increases the risk of head injury. Intramuscular glucagon may not work in alcohol-related hypoglycaemia, liver disease or prolonged hypoglycaemia.

21. Haemophilia

B. VIII

Haemophilia A is an X-linked recessive disorder of coagulation in which the patient cannot synthesise clotting factor VIII due to a gene mutation. Haemophilia B (a.k.a. Christmas disease) is caused by an inability to synthesise factor IX and is clinically indistinguishable from the much more common haemophilia A. Although usually familial (autosomal recessive) and more common in Ashkenazi Jews, a significant proportion of cases are caused by sporadic mutations. Factors VIII and IX are essential in the extrinsic clotting cascade, meaning that patients with haemophilia have a prolonged activated partial thromboplastin time ratio (aPTT). The intrinsic pathway does not require factors VIII or IX and is therefore unaffected by haemophilia – shown by a normal prothrombin time (PT). The bleeding time is also normal. Symptoms usually begin when the patient becomes mobile, i.e. when they begin to crawl or walk. Haemophiliacs typically suffer painful recurrent bleeds into the joints and soft tissues (haemarthrosis), which may eventually lead to crippling arthropathy and neuropathy.

The treatment of haemophilia A is with factor VIII concentrate either as a regular infusion or when actively bleeding. Patients receiving regular infusions have higher factor VIII levels and a better quality of life but are at higher risk of developing antibodies to the extrinsic factor VIII, which reduces its efficiency. Patients who receive factor VIII only when bleeding are less likely to form antibodies but are at increased risk of bleeding. Patients with mild disease may be treated with desmopressin (DDVAP), which releases factor VIII from internal stores. Factor VIII concentrate should be given prior to invasive procedures such as tooth extraction and surgery. Haemophilia B is treated with factor IX concentrate. It should be noted that many haemophiliacs who received blood products prior to the initiation of the blood screening programme have contracted blood-borne viruses such as HIV and hepatitis C.

Von Willebrand factor is a co-factor that binds to and mediates the actions of factor VIII binding to platelets. Inheritance is autosomal dominant in the majority and the gene is carried on chromosome 12. Replacement in severe disease involves cryoprecipitate or additional factor VIII.

Stephen Christmas was the first person described to have factor IX deficiency (1947–1993). He eventually died from acquired immune deficiency syndrome (AIDS), transmitted via a transfusion. The original case report of Christmas disease was reported in the Christmas edition of the *British Medical Journal* in 1952.

22. Gastrointestinal pathology

B. Crohn's disease

The clinical pictures of inflammatory bowel disease can often be very similar – classically a young woman with diarrhoea, pain and weight loss. Crohn's disease that is only located in the distal colon can appear indistinguishable from ulcerative colitis (UC) except on histology. The inflammation in Crohn's disease affects the entire thickness of the bowel wall – which is why it more often leads to complications such as fistulas and abscesses – whereas in UC the inflammation primarily affects the mucosa and submucosa leading to ulcer formation and crypt abscesses. Between ulcers, pseudopolyps can form, which tend to be very friable and easy to bleed. Differentiation in this case from gastrointestinal tuberculosis is difficult, but TB is more likely to produce caseating granulomas. However, in regions endemic with tuberculosis or in high-risk patients, a thorough history and high index of suspicion is required, even without the presence of caseating granulomas, and appropriate staining should be undertaken for histological specimens. Irritable bowel syndrome does not cause histological changes.

23. Blood film

B. Megaloblastic anaemia

Leucoerythroblastic anaemia describes the presence of immature cells – myelocytes and normoblasts – in the blood film. This can occur by any process that invades the bone marrow causing inappropriate release of immature cells into the circulation. This can be an infective process (such as tuberculous invasion of the bone marrow), primary bone marrow malignancy or metastatic spread into the marrow. Megaloblastic anaemia is an anaemia with a raised mean cell volume caused by a reduction in either folate or vitamin B_{12}.

24. Lung cancer

B. Metabolic alkalosis, small cell carcinoma

Small cell carcinoma comprises 20% of all lung cancers. Small cell lung carcinoma is known to metastasise early and is usually treated palliatively with chemotherapy (with a 80% mortality rate at 1 year). Patients with small cell carcinoma may present with symptoms of non-metastatic extrapulmonary manifestations such as endocrine syndromes (inappropriate ADH secretion and ectopic ACTH secretion). This patient presents <u>with a hypokalaemic metabolic alkalosis</u> <u>as a result of</u> <u>hypercortisolism associated with raised ACTH secretion</u> (this may also have caused her diabetes). <u>Hypokalaemia is responsible for myopathy</u>, as characterised by weakness in both lower limbs.

25. Cavernous sinus lesions

D. III, IV, VI and ophthalmic division of V

The cavernous sinus lies immediately posterior to the superior orbital fissure, and therefore those structures passing through the superior orbital fissure also pass through the cavernous sinus. Cranial nerve II (the optic nerve) passes through the optic foramen, medial and superior to the superior orbital fissure, and so does not run through the cavernous sinus. Those nerves that do are all of the nerves controlling eye movements (III, IV and VI), as well as the ophthalmic division of the V nerve (trigeminal) – this passes through the orbit to emerge from the supraorbital foramen as the supraorbital nerve and supply the skin of the forehead with sensory fibres. Clinically therefore, cavernous sinus pathology presents with a complete ophthalmoplegia of the affected side (often both sides are affected) and a loss of forehead sensation on the affected side. Causative pathologies include cavernous sinus thrombosis (often caused by spread of infection from the nasal and paranasal mucosa), meningioma, and, as the carotid artery runs through the cavernous sinus, carotid aneurysms and carotid-cavernous fistula. Because the cavernous sinuses of either side communicate with one another, thrombosis and fistula formation can cause symptoms on the other side as well. Often, the blocked venous drainage can cause local tissue oedema and proptosis, and carotid cavernous fistulae can give audible bruits in the orbital region.

Cavernous, from Latin *cavernosus* = cavity

26. Cognitive impairment (2)

D. Lewy body dementia

Frontotemporal dementia is very rare, and usually presents with personality change and disinhibition with a sparing of memory function early on in the disease. Of those with motor neuron disease, 5% also get frontotemporal dementia. Vascular dementia occurs with multiple transient ischaemic attacks (TIAs) and strokes, and while this patient is a smoker, there is no history of strokes or TIAs, and no neurological deficit on examination, suggestive of a stroke. Korsakoff psychosis is characterised by severe impairment of episodic memory function – patients are unable to form new episodic memories, and have impaired access to old episodic memories, and therefore are liable to confabulate. It is caused by mamillary body damage, normally secondary to untreated Wernicke encephalopathy, although it can be secondary to hypoxic brain damage or CNS infection. Depressive pseudodementia presents similarly to Alzheimer's disease, and is a common cause of misdiagnosis. It features depressed mood and anxiety, and lack of self-confidence can lead to an apparent short-term memory deficit, although with encouragement and close examination the memory deficit disappears.

Lewy body dementia is the second most common dementia after Alzheimer's disease. Characteristic features of Lewy body dementia include day-to-day fluctuating levels of cognitive functioning, visual hallucinations, sleep disturbance, transient loss of consciousness, recurrent falls and parkinsonian features (tremor, hypokinesia, rigidity and postural instability). Although people with Lewy body dementia are prone to hallucination, antipsychotics should be avoided as they precipitate severe parkinsonism in 60%. A Lewy body is an abnormality of the cytoplasm found within a neurone, containing various proteins and granular material. They are found in the cerebral cortex in patients with Lewy body dementia, and they are also found in patients with Parkinson's disease.

27. Complications of bone marrow transplant

B. Chronic graft-versus-host disease

Graft-versus-host disease can occur either acutely or chronically following any form of transplant. The severity can vary from self-limiting irritation to life-threatening disease. It occurs when transplanted immune cells build a reaction towards the host's cells. This can present with a myriad of symptoms but most commonly skin, liver and gastrointestinal tract manifestations. Treatment is twofold, symptomatic and immunosuppressive.

28. Diagnosis of abdominal pain (5)

A. Fitz-Hugh–Curtis syndrome

Fitz-Hugh–Curtis syndrome is a rare complication of pelvic inflammatory disease (PID), where ascending disease results in inflammation of the connective tissue around the liver (Glisson's capsule). It is often caused by gonococcal or chlamydial infection. It is predominantly a disease of women and only rarely affects men. Diagnosis is through the identification of pelvic inflammatory disease and the exclusion of other diseases including pancreatitis. Liver function tests are usually normal. Treatment is with antibiotics as for PID.

Thomas Fitz-Hugh Jr, American physician (1894-1963)

Arthur Curtis, American gynaecologist (1881-1955)

29. Diagnosis of cough (7)

D. *Pneumocystis jirovecii*

Pneumocystis jirovecii pneumonia is the most common AIDS-defining illness. In HIV-positive adults, the greatest risk factor for developing *Pneumocystis* pneumonia (PCP) is a CD4 count of below 200 cells/mm³. The incidence of PCP has reduced significantly with the use of highly active antiretroviral therapy (HAART) and routine primary prophylaxis in those with a CD4 count of less than 200 cells/mm³. Most cases of PCP occurs in patients who are unaware of their HIV infection, or do not use HAART or PCP prophylaxis due to intolerance or non-compliance. PCP could also affect patients who are on chronic immunosuppressive therapy, solid organ transplant recipients and bone marrow transplant recipients. Patients present with a non-productive dry cough, dyspnoea, weight loss, fatigue and possibly pleuritic chest pain, which is uncommon in PCP without a pneumothorax. Chest examination is usually unremarkable. Chest X-ray findings include bilateral symmetrical interstitial infiltrates with perihilar reticular opacities, lobar consolidation, nodular lesions, pneumothorax and pneumomediastinum, although it can be normal. The treatment involves trimethoprim/sulfamethoxazole (TMP/SMX), and corticosteroids in severe cases. Patients with respiratory compromise require admission to the intensive care unit for mechanical ventilation.

30. Palpitations (2)

E. Phaeochromocytoma

Phaeochromocytoma is a rare tumour arising from the catecholamine-producing chromaffin cells from the adrenal medulla. Approximately 90% arise in the adrenal gland and the remainder are extra-adrenal in origin. Most of these tumours are sporadic in origin but about 10% are part of manifestation of a hereditary syndrome such as multiple endocrine neoplasia type 2, Von Hippel–Lindau syndrome and neurofibromatosis. The patient presents with palpitations, headache, excessive sweating, pallor and paroxysmal hypertension. Some present with a complication of hypertension, e.g. stroke, myocardial infarction, hypertensive retinopathy and accelerated phase hypertension. The diagnosis is obtained by increased levels of urinary cathecholamines, metanephrines and normetanephrines. Treatment options include medical management, which aims to block the effects of catecholamine excess by controlling hypertension using alpha receptor blockers, or surgical removal of the tumour.

31. Diagnosis of neurological dysfunction (3)

D. Subacute combined degeneration of the cord

This patient appears to be isolated and quite likely living near to poverty (despite assumedly having come to the UK to escape as much). There is a possibility that various health issues have not come to light. The patient has not admitted to known HIV, but she comes from a high-risk area and she may be disguising it or in denial. She does not appear to be taking medication for HIV, and a polyneuropathy is more commonly secondary to highly active antiretroviral therapy (HAART) (nucleoside reverse transcriptase analogues (NRTIs), in particular didanosine and stavudine). She denies diabetes, and occult type II diabetes seems unlikely in view of her nutritional status.

Concerning the pattern of the weakness and sensory loss, the weakness appears to be mixed, in that there are brisk knee jerks and upgoing plantars indicating an upper motor neuron lesion (located in the spinal cord as the legs are involved symmetrically and the arms not at all), but there are absent ankle jerks. The sensory loss appears to be of the peripheral polyneuropathological type. The spinal cord involvement rules out Guillain–Barré syndrome (as does the slow onset not progressing to involve the upper limbs); it also rules out either HIV-related or diabetic polyneuropathy. Tabes dorsalis affects the posterior columns rather than the corticospinal tract, therefore subacute combined degeneration of the cord is the answer.

Subacute combined degeneration of the cord is caused by vitamin B_{12} deficiency. Her likely malnourishment and poverty explains this, which could be exacerbated by, for example, tapeworm infection. Note the conjunctival pallor – B_{12} deficiency also causes macrocytic anaemia. The pathology is demyelination, and this can affect the corticospinal tract (predominantly lower down), posterior columns, and peripheral nerves, variably. The picture of a subacute onset of mixed upper and lower motor neuron lower limb weakness is classical.

32. Diagnosis of skin lesions (2)

C. Irregular pigment network

Erythema of the border when looking at a pigmented lesion can raise suspicion that it may be malignant melanoma, however seborrhoeic keratoses can become inflamed and this is therefore non-specific. A granular surface is a typical feature of seborrhoeic keratoses when inspected up close. A "stuck-on" appearance is again typical for seborrhoeic keratoses and does not require dermoscopy to spot. Telangiectasia of the skin surface is far more typical of basal cell carcinomas. An irregular pigment network may be highly important in differentiating a malignant melanoma from a benign pigmented lesion, and may be picked up by dermoscopy – a flat low-resolution glass is placed directly on the area of interest to magnify the appearance of the skin.

33. Malignant melanoma (2)

D. Invasive depth

The risk of recurrence of malignant melanoma has a lot to do with how deep the lesion has invaded, as measured by the Breslow thickness: Depth <0.76 mm = low risk, 0.76–1.5 mm = medium risk, >1.5 mm = high risk. Staging also depends upon the thickness: Stage 1 has tumour <2 mm, stage 2 >2 mm (stage 3 has lymph node involvement, stage 4 has one or more metastases). Colour, diameter and weight do not give information on prognosis, and grade may do but less so than the Breslow thickness.

Alexander Breslow, American pathologist (1928-1980)

34. Electrocardiogram (5)

B. Check the drug chart for possible causes

Tricyclic antidepressants (e.g. imipramine, amitriptyline), type 1a anti-arrhythmics (e.g. quinidine, procainamide) and hypokalaemia are known to cause torsade de pointes. This condition is significant in that it can lead to ventricular fibrillation and therefore needs to be treated. Diuretics are a common cause of hypokalaemia. Between reviewing the drug chart and looking up this patient's most recent serum potassium, you would be wise to inform your seniors and a cardiologist. The patient should be linked to a cardiac monitor. It would be wise to ensure the crash trolley is ready for use.

35. Diagnosis of chest infection (1)

E. Severe community-acquired pneumonia

There is no history of choking or aspiration or any at risk conditions (e.g. epileptic fits, Parkinson's disease, alcoholism) to suggest aspiration pneumonia. Whilst the blunting of the costophrenic angle suggests an effusion, it sounds small and is unlikely to represent an empyema – it could be a parapneumonic effusion or could be unrelated. Whilst he was in hospital for a hernia repair, this was likely a short visit and it was 2 months ago, after which he has been well, so it is not hospital-acquired pneumonia. Community-acquired pneumonia is graded using the CURB-65 score: patients score from 0 to 5, picking up points for: 1) confusion (new AMTS <8), 2) urea >7 mmol/L, 3) respiratory rate >30/min, 4) blood pressure <90 systolic or <60 diastolic mmHg, or 5) age >65. A score of 0–1 is mild, 2 is moderate, and 3 or more is severe. Our patient scored at least 3 for his age, new confusion and a respiratory rate >30 so has a severe community-acquired pneumonia. Hospital guidelines for antibiotic use in pneumonia vary across the country due to differing organisms and sensitivities, but severity of pneumonia and the community/hospital distinction are used to guide initial empirical therapies.

36. Emergency management (1)

B. Intramuscular benzylpenicillin and call ambulance

This patient has the clinical features of meningitis with septicaemia (neck stiffness in association with general illness and a non-blanching purpuric rash). It is essential that this patient is given antibiotics as soon as possible and admitted to a high-dependency unit. If the patient is seen in the community, she should be given an intramuscular dose of benzylpenicillin whilst transport to hospital is being arranged. Once in hospital, the patient will require intravenous antibiotics (e.g. cefotaxime) for at least 7 days in addition to supportive measures.

37. Investigation of shortness of breath (2)

D. Spirometry

With his history of smoking, it is highly likely that this patient has developed chronic obstructive pulmonary disease (COPD). The diagnosis of COPD requires spirometry. A post-bronchodilator FEV_1 of <80% of the predicted value and FEV_1/FVC <70% confirms the diagnosis. A low peak flow is consistent with COPD, but it is not a specific test as it could underestimate the severity of airflow obstruction and is unable to differentiate obstructive and restrictive disorders. Chest X-ray is useful in excluding other lung pathology and might detect bullae associated with COPD.

38. Diagnosis of chest pain (3)

B. Gastro-oesophageal reflux disease

Differentiating gastro-oesophageal reflux disease (GORD) from a cardiac cause of pain can be extremely difficult. In this case the salient features are that the pain occurs on lying down to go to sleep. Although in unstable angina this may occur, you would also expect a patient to report pain on increased exertion as well. A GTN spray may relieve both GORD and angina as the nitrates cause smooth muscle relaxation in the oesophagus as well as coronary arteries.

GORD is associated with obesity, smoking, alcohol, hernias and pregnancy. Patients generally present with intermittent pain, or heartburn, which may be related to lifestyle factors such as large meals or alcohol. Medications can also contribute and should be reviewed. Endoscopy is not usually indicated for the diagnosis in young, otherwise healthy, patients, however urgent referrals should be considered in anyone over the age of 55 with new-onset symptoms or warning signs of weight loss, gastrointestinal (GI) bleeding or anaemia. Management of dyspepsia is by modification of lifestyle factors including weight loss, and pharmacological treatment with proton pump inhibitors. Complications of longstanding reflux are the development of Barrett's oesophagus and the formation of strictures.

39. Hypoxia

A. Check her fluid balance chart

This woman is probably suffering from pulmonary oedema, which is easily caused or exacerbated by overadministration of intravenous fluids, and she will become even more vulnerable to hospital-acquired pneumonia. At such low saturations, an arterial blood gas analysis should be undertaken as it is superior to pulse oximetry (which can be erroneous at low saturations) and will also allow you to monitor carbon dioxide levels and renal compensation. Whilst pneumonia and pulmonary embolism (PE) are possible diagnoses, it only takes seconds to review her fluid balance chart.

40. Management of hypothermia

C. Intravenous lorazepam

Myxoedema coma is a rare presentation of extreme hypothyroidism. It is a medical emergency and treatment should be initiated before confirmation of the diagnosis. Patients present with a depressed level of consciousness, low body temperature and convulsions. An intravenous bolus of triiodothyronine (T_3) is given. Warm blankets could be used to increase body temperature. The thyroid failure should be assumed to be secondary to hypothalamus or pituitary disease and IV hydrocortisone should be given before thyroid function tests become available. High-flow oxygen is given to patients with low oxygen saturations.

41. Diagnosis of diabetes

B. HbA1C level

In patients with presenting symptoms suggesting diabetes mellitus, the diagnosis could be confirmed by fasting glucose $\geq$7.0 mmol/L or random glucose $\geq$11.1 mmol/L. In asymptomatic patients, two samples are required to confirm diabetes. Urine is tested for glucose and ketones. An oral glucose tolerance test is indicated when fasting plasma glucose is within 6.1–6.9 mmol/L or random plasma glucose within 7.8–11.0 mmol/L (levels suggestive of impaired glucose tolerance). HbA1C is not used for diagnosis but is rather used as a measure of glycaemic control over a period of months.

42. Medication review

B. Atenolol

Clopidogrel prevents platelets forming a thrombus, however its effects can last for 7 days so you should keep an eye out for all patients on clopidogrel destined for surgery and ensure an alternative anticoagulation treatment is given 7 days prior to intervention. It should be noted that: 1) beta-blockers are contraindicated in asthma, a very common co-morbidity; 2) beta-adrenergic receptors stimulate the fight-or-flight response; 3) beta-1 receptors increase cardiac contractility, heart rate and renin release; 4) beta-2 receptors relax (bronchial) smooth muscle (the target of salbutamol); and 5) beta-3 receptors instigate lipolysis in adipose tissue. Atenolol is more selective in blocking beta-1 receptors and patients with asthma should be given calcium-channel blockers like diltiazem instead.

43. Side effects of methotrexate

B. Alcohol should be absolutely avoided whilst taking methotrexate

A baseline chest X-ray is indeed taken when starting methotrexate – pulmonary fibrosis can be a side effect of long-term methotrexate use. Liver function aberrations are the most common side effect and can lead to hepatic fibrosis soon after starting methotrexate. Therefore, liver function tests are initially monitored weekly, followed by fortnightly then every 4–6 weeks. Whilst alcohol intake above 12 units per week can increase the risk of liver damage, it is permissible for patients to have a small amount of alcohol, though it is advised against. Neutropenia and myelosuppression are risks and therefore the full blood count is monitored along with liver function tests. Methotrexate blocks the action of folate and therefore pregnancy is contraindicated due to the risk of neural tube defects.

44. Raised intracranial pressure

E. Transient bilateral visual loss

Jaw claudication is a sign of temporal arteritis (moving jaw contracts the temporalis muscle and thus irritates the inflamed temporal artery). Kernig's sign (with the patient lying on their back with their hip flexed, and the knee extension causing pain) is a sign of meningism as the manoeuvre stretches the nerve roots in the leg, whose sheaths are continuous with the meninges of the central nervous system. On lying down, gravity causes an increase in intracranial pressure so it would be expected that the symptoms would get worse. Increased intracranial pressure could either cause, or be caused by, hydrocephalus, and this can compress the optic nerve (increased fluid in the nerve sheath). A late sign therefore may be episodes of transient bilateral visual loss, provoked by postural change, e.g. lying down. Fundoscopy should be conducted, looking for papilloedema. Finally, as increased intracranial pressure is considered, lumbar puncture is contraindicated as it may provoke transforaminal herniation and thus cardiorespiratory compromise by medullary compression.

45. Bronchial carcinoma

D. Squamous cell carcinoma

Lung carcinoma is the most common cause of cancer death in men and women in the UK. It is strongly associated with cigarette smoking. Cigarette smoking is thought to be responsible for more than 90% of cases of lung carcinoma. Squamous cell carcinoma is the most common histological type, which accounts for about 35% of the bronchial carcinoma. Patients with hypercalcaemia are most likely to have squamous cell carcinoma as it stimulates the secretion of parathyroid hormone-like peptides, which causes a rise in blood calcium levels by osteolysis in bone and promoting the reabsorption of calcium from renal tubules.

46. Neurological dysfunction

C. Median nerve

The nerve roots can be ruled out, as C6 supplies the thumb and index finger, and C8 supplies the fourth and little finger. The ulnar nerve enters the hand near the ulna and supplies sensation to the medial half of the fourth finger and the entire fifth finger. The radial nerve supplies sensation to a patch of skin on the radial side of the back of the hand, and very little of the fingers if any (there are individual variations). The sensory distribution described is supplied by the median nerve. The thenar muscles are supplied by the median nerve, hence the thenar wasting and weakness of thumb abduction (abductor pollicis brevis). The shooting pains and lack of any history of trauma would make carpal tunnel syndrome the most likely cause.

Carpal tunnel syndrome is more common in women, during pregnancy and with certain medical conditions such as rheumatoid arthritis, acromegaly and hypothyroidism. Patients experience tingling and numbness in the radial three and a half digits, which may be followed by wasting of the thenar eminence (supplied by the median nerve). Clinical tests that help confirm carpal tunnel syndrome include Tinel's test (tapping over the median nerve at the wrist reproduces symptoms) and Phalen's test (symptoms are reproduced by holding the wrist palmarflexed for 1 minute).

Jules Tinel, French neurologist (1879-1952)

George Phalen, American orthopaedic surgeon (1911-1998)

47. Diagnosis of rheumatoid arthritis (1)

E. Ulnar deviation of one or more fingers for more than 6 weeks

All of the above clinical features are suggestive of rheumatoid arthritis, the important difference however is that ulnar deviation of the fingers is a late manifestation that occurs due to subluxation at the metacarpophalangeal joints, which only happens after significant irreversible joint damage. Ideally any diagnostic criteria would focus on diagnosing early so that disease-modifying anti-rheumatic drugs (DMARDs) can be started promptly. Rheumatoid arthritis commonly causes morning stiffness (in osteoarthritis stiffness is typically worse after movement at the affected joints), and due to the systemic nature of the cause, diffuse and sometimes symmetrical joint involvement can be seen, whereas osteoarthritis is commonly related to physical wear and tear and thus can be localised and is not necessarily symmetrical.

The diagnosis of rheumatoid arthritis is made using the American Rheumatism Association criteria, requiring four of the following seven factors to be present:

1. Morning stiffness >1 hour for more than 6 weeks
2. Arthritis of hand joints (wrist, MCP, PIP) for more than 6 weeks
3. Arthritis of three or more joint areas for more than 6 weeks
4. Symmetric arthritis for more than 6 weeks
5. Rheumatoid nodules
6. Characteristic X-ray findings
7. Positive rheumatoid factor

The four characteristic X-ray findings of rheumatoid arthritis are soft tissue swelling, narrowed joint space, juxta-articular erosions and subluxation.

48. Statistics (2)

D. 83%

The specificity is the ability of an investigation to detect a truly negative test result.

Specificity = number of true negatives / (number of true negatives + number of false positives) × 100

In this case = 25 (25 + 5) × 100 = 83%

49. Sepsis syndromes

D. Severe sepsis

Septicaemia describes the state of having an organism in the blood, which this woman has; however this does not fully describe the situation. Systemic inflammatory response syndrome (SIRS) is defined as having two or more of the following four criteria: pulse >90, temperature <36°C/>38°C, Respiratory rate >20/PaCO$_2$ <4.3 (hyperventilatory hypocapnia), or white cell count <4/>12. This woman has SIRS as evidenced by her pulse, temperature and respiratory rate. The combination of SIRS and septicaemia is known as sepsis. Severe sepsis is when a septic patient is showing signs of organ hypoperfusion – for instance, oliguria (kidney hypoperfusion), confusion (brain hypoperfusion) or serum lactate >4 (muscle hypoperfusion). This woman is oliguric and confused. Shock means hypotension, and septic shock is defined as sepsis with refractory hypotension (i.e. hypotension persevering in spite of fluid resuscitation), which does not apply to this patient, therefore she is best described as having severe sepsis. This may indicate that present antibiotic therapy is inadequate and that aggressive intravenous fluid resuscitation should be instituted.

50. Nephrotic syndrome

D. >3.5 g of protein lost in the urine over 24 hours

Nephrotic syndrome is a triad of proteinuria, hypoalbuminaemia and oedema. The proteinuria is classically quantified as more than 3.5 g in 24 hours. When phaeochromocytoma is suspected, 72-hour urine collection is performed to look for urinary metanephrines and other catecholamine metabolites. Quantification of proteinuria, rather than simply dipstick testing, is important as both hypoalbuminaemia and proteinuria are non-specific and can be present in important clinical differentials (cardiac failure can feature mild proteinuria, and liver failure can result in hypoalbuminaemia – both cause oedema and fatigue). A newer test that can spare the hassle of 24-hour urine collection is the urine protein:creatinine ratio, which can reliably predict the amount of protein excreted in urine over 24 hours from a random urine sample. Nephrotic syndrome is most commonly caused by glomerulonephritides, and so further testing should look for other features of glomerulonephritis and causes thereof (renal autoimmune screen, serum and urine electrophoresis, urine microscopy). Adults with nephrotic syndrome should all get a renal biopsy to further elucidate the cause; in children, minimal change glomerulonephritis is the most common cause, and this normally reverses with steroids, hence biopsy can be avoided unless there are other concerning features or there is little response to steroids.

Practice Paper 6: Questions

1. Amenorrhoea

A 16-year-old female attends her GP complaining of a persistent lack of periods. She has a short stature, low-set ears and broad square-shaped chest. She has a short fourth metacarpal. There is radio-radial delay on examination.

What would the most appropriate diagnostic test be in this case?

A Growth hormone level
B Karyotype analysis
C Magnetic resonance angiography
D Thyroid function test
E Ultrasound of the ovaries

2. Myasthenia gravis

Which of the following investigation findings would you NOT expect in myasthenia gravis?

A Decrementing response on electromyography
B Hyperplasia of the thymus gland or thymoma on computed tomography (CT) of the chest
C Positive acetylcholine receptor antibodies
D Rimmed vacuoles on muscle biopsy
E Tensilon test reduces weakness

3. Hyperkalaemia

A 78-year-old man admitted with severe sepsis secondary to a chest infection develops worsening acute renal failure. An arterial blood gas reading, other than showing metabolic acidosis, also reveals a potassium level of 7.2 mmol/L. You ask the nurse for an electrocardiogram (ECG).

Which of the following changes is NOT associated with hyperkalaemia?

A Broadening of the QRS complex
B Deepening Q-waves
C Flattening of the P-waves
D Tented T-waves
E Ventricular fibrillation

4. Myocardial infarction

A 75-year-old man with known heart failure is likely to have had a myocardial infarction. He is now haemodynamically stable on the ward. A 12-hour troponin level is raised.

Which investigation will confirm your diagnosis?

A 24-hour ECG
B Exercise ECG
C Troponin level at 48 hours
D Nuclear studies of the myocardium
E None of the above

5. Pruritus

A 45-year-old woman presents with a 5-month history of worsening generalised itching. There is nothing remarkable in the woman's medical history and there is no sign of any skin lesion or inflammatory disorder of the skin. You take some blood tests for a pruritus screen.

Which of the following tests would NOT reveal a cause for pruritus and thus is not indicated?

A Electrolytes
B Full blood count
C Iron studies
D Thyroid function tests
E Urea

6. Seizures

Which of the following symptoms would NOT be caused by complex partial seizures?

A Déjà-vu
B Fumbling or rubbing, slightly odd limb movements
C Shooting/electric shock-like pains in the limbs
D Smell and/or taste hallucinations
E Subtly impaired conscious level

7. Spinal cord compression

A 70-year-old woman with a background of bowel cancer, which was resected 2 years ago, presents with a 3-week history of back pain, progressive clumsiness and heaviness of the legs with paraesthesia. On examination, the arms are normal, but there is weakness throughout the legs, brisk reflexes, upgoing plantars and diminished sensation bilaterally up to the belly button.

Where is the lesion likely to be?

A C5
B L2
C T8
D T10
E T12

8. Sepsis

A 50-year-old man being treated for inoperable gastric cancer with chemotherapy presents with a sore throat and cough. On examination, he has a temperature of 38.2°C.

Which of the following statements indicates the most severe life-threatening illness?

A Cough of >2 weeks duration
B Neutrophils $>15 \times 10^9$/L
C Neutrophils $<0.5 \times 10^9$/L
D Severe vomiting
E Weight loss

9. Radiographic changes in ankylosing spondylitis

A 22-year-old man with a family history of psoriasis attends clinic complaining of lower back and buttock pains on and off for the past 6 months. This is worse in the mornings and associated with stiffness.

Which of the following findings on magnetic resonance imaging (MRI) would be first to appear and thus diagnostic of early ankylosing spondylitis?

A Bamboo spine
B Fusion of the sacroiliac joints
C Osteophyte formation
D Sacroiliitis
E Syndesmophyte formation

10. Management of toxicity

An 80-year-old woman is admitted to hospital with a right neck of femur fracture. She was found to become drowsy with a respiratory rate of 8/min after a dose of intravenous morphine. There are pinpoint pupils on examination

What should you do?

A Give intravenous flumazenil
B Give intravenous magnesium sulphate
C Give intravenous N-acetylcysteine
D Give intravenous naloxone
E Give intravenous sodium bicarbonate

11. Squamous cell carcinoma

Which of the following statements is FALSE about squamous cell carcinoma?

A Curettage is the first line of management
B Sun exposure is a risk factor
C They are ill-defined lesions and often ulcerate
D They are more common in kidney transplant patients
E They can metastasise to lymph nodes

12. Management of urinary tract infection

A 28-year-old pregnant woman has a routine mid-stream urine sample taken for dipstick testing and microscopy culture and sensitivities. She is asymptomatic.

Which of the following results does not warrant a course of antibiotics?

A All of the results below require treatment
B Leukocyte esterase negative, nitrites negative, but $>10^5$/ml Gram-negative rods on microscopy
C Leukocyte esterase negative, nitrites positive
D Leukocyte esterase positive, nitrites negative
E Leukocyte esterase positive, nitrites positive

13. Side effects of anti-tuberculous medication

A 35-year-old homeless man diagnosed with new tuberculosis 1 month previously and started on treatment presents with a loss of colour vision.

Which of the following medications is responsible?

A Ethambutol
B Isoniazid
C Pyrazinamide
D Rifampicin
E Streptomycin

14. Hypothyroidism

A 64-year-old woman with known heart disease presents to her GP with weight gain, weakness and bilateral leg swelling. On examination she has slow-relaxing elbow reflexes. Thyroid function tests show an elevated TSH and low serum T_4 level.

Which of the following medications might be contributing to her symptoms?

A Amiodarone
B Fluoxetine
C Lisinopril
D Prednisolone
E Simvastatin

15. Painful fingers

A 52-year-old woman presents with a 2-year history of painful fingers. In cold weather her fingers turn pale and then through blue to red, at which point she experiences severe pain in the fingers. Over the last few months, she has had some retrosternal pain on eating and experiences some reflux. On examination the fingers appear to be swollen and tense, with some dilated nail-fold capillary loops and a small crusted ulcer is present on a fingertip.

What is the most likely diagnosis?

A Dermatomyositis
B Limited cutaneous systemic sclerosis
C Primary Raynaud phenomenon
D Sarcoid
E Systemic lupus erythematosus

16. Palpitations (3)

A 26-year-old woman presents to the GP with a history of palpitations. She also feels hot most of the time and has noticed some weight loss. On examination, she has a "startled" look with lid lag and lid retraction. There is a palpable neck lump on examination that moves up on swallowing.

Which of the following investigations will be LEAST appropriate?

A 24-hour electrocardiogram
B Technetium-99 scintigraphy
C Fine-needle aspiration
D Thyroid function tests
E TSH-receptor antibodies

17. Haemoptysis (2)

A 15-year-old boy has recently started coughing up blood. He has had a non-productive cough for about 6 months with intermittent haemoptysis. Otherwise he is normally fit and well. On examination, finger clubbing is noted. Chest examination reveals basal crepitations with reduced air entry. Pulmonary function tests reveal a raised transfer factor. A blood test shows low haemoglobin, low mean cell volume, low iron and low ferritin. Autoantibody profiling is negative.

What is the most likely diagnosis?

A Goodpasture syndrome
B Idiopathic pulmonary haemosiderosis
C Microscopic polyarteritis
D Systemic lupus erythromatosus
E Wegener granulomatosis

18. Antibody testing

A 64-year-old woman presents with a 3-week history of progressive painless haematuria, hypertension, breathlessness and haemoptysis. There is no evidence of epistaxis. Her blood pressure is now 190/110 mmHg, and her chest X-ray shows haemorrhagic pulmonary infiltrates in the lower zones. Her bloods reveal a creatinine level of 340 µmol/L and a raised C-reactive protein.

Which of the following antibody tests would confirm the likely diagnosis?

A Anti-double-stranded DNA antibodies (anti-dsDNA)
B Anti-glomerular basement membrane antibodies (anti-GBM)
C Anti-ribonucleoprotein antibodies (anti-RNP)
D Cytoplasmic anti-neutrophil cytoplasm antibodies (cANCA)
E Perinuclear anti-neutrophil cytoplasm antibodies (pANCA)

19. Management of shortness of breath (4)

A 60-year-old man presents to the emergency department with progressive breathlessness on exertion. He has a past medical history of hypertension, diabetes mellitus and chronic obstructive pulmonary disease. He has also complained of weight loss for the past 6 months. On examination, he was alert with a respiratory rate of 25/min and an oxygen saturation reading of 86% in air. He has distended neck veins, facial oedema and bilateral arm swelling.

Which of the following management options is NOT appropriate initially?

A Consider intravenous dexamethasone and radiotherapy
B Consider intubation if in respiratory compromise
C Consider percutaneous endovascular stenting
D Give oxygen to maintain oxygen saturation at 88–92%
E Request a chest X-ray

20. Atrial fibrillation

Which of the following is NOT a cause for atrial fibrillation?

A Abdominal aortic aneurysm
B Acute infection
C Binge drinking
D Hypertension
E Idiopathic

21. Blood groups

Which of the following is the universal recipient in blood transfusion?

A A+
B AB–
C AB+

D B–
E O

22. Generalised weakness

A 43-year-old woman presents to the GP with generalised weakness. She notices that she has been gaining weight for the past 3 months despite a normal diet. She has a past medical history of asthma, which is poorly controlled, and she was admitted to the hospital twice last year due to exacerbations. On examination, her blood pressure is 160/90 mmHg. She has bruises on both shins, with wasting and weakness of her proximal thigh muscles.

Which of the following is the most likely diagnosis?

A Addison's disease
B Cushing's syndrome
C Hypothyroidism
D Hyperthyroidism
E Hypercalcaemia

23. Investigation of jaundice

A 25-year-old female student, who is normally fit and well, presents to the emergency department 3 weeks before her final exams. She is drowsy and confused. On examination, she has a hepatic flap and is jaundiced. There is also tender hepatomegaly.

Which of the following is a pertinent first-line investigation?

A Ferritin levels
B Gamma-glutamyl transferase (GGT)
C Hepatitis screen
D Lumbar puncture
E Paracetamol levels

24. Management of skin conditions

An 83-year-old woman who lives in a care home presents with a 2-week history of itching. A few of the other residents have since complained of similar symptoms. You suspect scabies.

Which of the following statements about scabies is FALSE?

A All clothes, bedsheets and any upholstery contacted by the patient should be washed thoroughly
B Burrows are often in web spaces of the digits, wrists, elbows, and male genitals
C Diagnosis is by examining scraped-off burrows under a microscope
D Treatment is application of topical malathion or permethrin
E Treatment with topical agents can be one-off or can ideally be repeated 7 days later

25. Investigation of muscle weakness

A 35-year-old woman presents with a history of weakness and paraesthesia for 2 weeks. It started with some unusual sensations in her feet and hands, then some days later she noticed her feet were dragging as she walked. Then over the next week she became unable to get out of her chair and developed arm weakness. She says she had some diarrhoea and abdominal cramps around 4 weeks ago. On examination there is weakness throughout the legs and arms in a patchy distribution varying between grades 2 and 4, reflexes are diminished throughout, and there is reduced sensation in the feet up to mid-shin level.

Which of the following investigation findings is suggestive of the likely diagnosis?

A Multifocal decreased motor conduction block only
B Multifocal decreased motor conduction speed with/without conduction block
C Oligoclonal bands on lumbar puncture
D Positive antiviral or antibacterial antibodies to campylobacter
E Raised lymphocytes on lumbar puncture

26. Hepatitis serology

A 45-year-old woman presents with malaise, joint pains and jaundice. A hepatitis screen is sent and returns with the following results:

Hepatitis B surface antigen (HBsAg) – POSITIVE
Hepatitis B 'e' antigen (HBeAg) – POSITIVE
Hepatitis B core antibody (HBcAb) – POSITIVE

Which of the following is the most likely diagnosis?

A Acute hepatitis B infection
B Chronic hepatitis B infection
C Hepatitis B immunity following previous infection
D Hepatitis B immunity following previous vaccination
E No hepatitis B infection

27. Lumbar puncture

A lumbar puncture in a patient with headache shows the following results:

Cells	460/mm³ (normal range <4/mm³)
Predominant cell type	Lymphocytes
Glucose	1.3 mmol/L (normal range 2–9 mmol/L)
Protein	1200 mg/L (normal range 200–400 mg/L)

India ink staining after the culture is negative

Which one of the following are these findings consistent with?

A Bacterial meningitis
B Cryptococcal meningitis
C Malignant meningitis
D Tubercular meningitis
E Viral meningitis

28. Management of hyperkalaemia

Which of the following medications used in the management of severe hyperkalaemia does not actually lower serum potassium, but rather is cardioprotective by acting as a membrane stabiliser?

A Calcium gluconate
B Calcium resonium
C Dextrose 50% with Actrapid insulin
D Furosemide
E Salbutamol

29. Management of hypertension

A 60-year-old man with known type 1 diabetes mellitus for the past 20 years has come to his GP for his annual diabetic check. His blood pressure is 160/90 mmHg today. He is found to have a urinary albumin/creatinine ratio (ACR) of >2.5 mg/mmol, suggestive of microalbuminuria.

Which of the following drugs is proven to reduce microalbuminuria?

A ACE inhibitors
B Alpha-blockers
C Beta-blockers
D Calcium channel blockers
E Thiazide

30. Malabsorption

An 18-year-old female is newly diagnosed with coeliac disease following a prolonged history of diarrhoea, malaise and weight loss.

Which of the following is the most suitable initial management?

A Exclusion of gluten from the diet
B Exclusion of lactose from diet
C Immunosuppressive agents
D Non-steroidal anti-inflammatories
E Stool-forming drugs such as loperamide

31. Brain tumours

Which of the following patients is most likely to have a cerebellopontine angle tumour?

A A 30-year-old woman with unilateral lower motor neuron facial weakness progressing over days and covered in café au lait spots

B A 40-year-old woman with insidious onset unilateral deafness, on Weber's testing sound is louder ipsilaterally

C A 50-year-old man with bilateral facial weakness, nasal voice and swallowing difficulty progressing over 3 months

D A 50-year-old woman with insidious-onset unilateral deafness, on Weber's testing sound is louder contralaterally, and with some ipsilateral reduced facial sensation

E A 65-year-old man with insidious-onset mild bilateral sensorineural deafness and no other neurological abnormality

32. Chest injury

An 85-year-old retired soldier defends a young woman from being mugged, only to find himself stabbed in the left side of the chest.

On arrival at the emergency department, which of the following features would be most relevant?

A Beck's triad

B Kussmaul breathing

C Kussmaul's sign

D Virchow's triad

E Witnessed Stokes–Adams attack

33. Complications of hepatitis infection

A 68-year-old man with chronic hepatitis B virus infection presents with a 1-month history of weight loss, malaise and right upper quadrant discomfort. On examination he has mild ascites and appears cachectic.

What is the most likely diagnosis?

A Cholangiocarcinoma

B Cirrhosis of the liver

C Hepatocellular carcinoma

D Reactivation of hepatitis B

E Right-heart failure

34. Conn's syndrome

You have been asked to explain the causes of hypertension to a patient recently diagnosed with Conn's syndrome.

Which of the following is an incorrect statement that should NOT feature in your explanation?

A Angiotensin I is converted to angiotensin II mainly in the lungs

B Angiotensin II causes blood pressure to rise but will be low in this patient

C Conn's syndrome causes excess aldosterone, the vasoconstriction from which leads to hypertension

D Hypertensive patients are often vulnerable to hypokalaemia as a side effect of their medication

E The patient is vulnerable to hypokalaemia as they are excreting too much in their urine

35. Dysphagia

An 88-year-old man presents with a month-long history of difficulty swallowing solids. He has noticed his clothes are looser on him now and he has a significant smoking history.

What is the most likely diagnosis?

A Achalasia

B Lung carcinoma

C Motor neurone disease

D Oesophageal *Candida*

E Oesophageal carcinoma

36. Diagnosis of chest infection (2)

A 71-year-old woman is admitted with 5 days of cough productive of purulent sputum and fevers, which has not improved with oral antibiotics prescribed by the GP. She is now confused and dehydrated with some renal impairment evident from the bloods (urea 9 mmol/L, creatinine 140 µmol/L). Chest X-ray now shows bilateral consolidation.

Urinary antigen testing should be done looking for which causative pathogen?

A *Escherichia coli*

B *Haemophilus influenza*

C *Legionella* spp.

D *Mycoplasma pneumoniae*

E Viruses

37. Diagnosis of cough (8)

A 40-year-old man presents to the GP with a cough. His cough has been present for about 2 months, and it has become worse over the past few weeks. Besides that, he also finds himself easily becoming short of breath when he exercises. The cough is dry and non-productive. He does not produce any blood-tinged sputum. He has not lost weight, never smokes and has no other significant past medical history.

What is the most likely diagnosis?

A Asthma
B Chronic obstructive pulmonary disease
C Interstitial pulmonary fibrosis
D Lung cancer
E Pneumonia

38. Diagnosis of Cushing's syndrome

A 40-year-old woman presents to the GP with generalised weakness and weight loss. She noticed that she had become more tanned despite not travelling abroad. On examination, there were bruises on both of her shins. A provisional diagnosis of Cushing's syndrome is made.

Which of the following test is NOT helpful in this case?

A 48-hour high-dose dexamethasone suppression test
B Computed tomography (CT) of the adrenals
C CT of the chest
D Overnight low-dose dexamethasone suppression test
E Plasma ACTH

39. Diagnosis of neurological dysfunction (4)

A 55-year-old man presents with 6 months of progressive weakness in his arms and legs. On further questioning he reveals that he has choked quite a few times recently on swallowing liquids. He is a smoker but has no significant past medical history. He is British and has not travelled widely. On examination of the cranial nerves, his palate does not rise much on the left on saying "aah", and does not rise on the right at all. On examination of his arms, there is wasting of the dorsal interosseous muscles and fasciculations in the right forearm and left deltoid, there is diffuse weakness (grade 4), the reflexes are present or brisk, and there is no sensory deficit. On examination of the legs, there are fasciculations seen in the thighs, some proximal weakness on the left, and brisk knee jerks and upgoing plantar reflexes. Again there is no sensory deficit.

Which of the following diagnoses is most likely?

A Cervical spondylosis
B HIV-related motor neurone disease-like syndrome
C Motor neurone disease
D Multiple sclerosis
E Syringomyelia and syringobulbia

40. Diagnosis of rheumatoid arthritis (2)

A 43-year-old woman presents with a history of 5 months of symmetrical hand pain and swelling with morning stiffness. You suspect rheumatoid arthritis.

Which of the following tests is the most sensitive and specific for rheumatoid arthritis?

A ANCA
B Anti-CCP antibodies
C Anti-centromere antibodies
D Rheumatoid factor
E Soft tissue swelling and bony erosions on X-ray of the hands

41. Diagnosis of skin lesions (3)

A 55-year-old woman presents with a 4-month history of an erythematous rash over her cheeks, nose and forehead. There appears to be multiple small papules and a few pustules on a background of erythematous skin.

What is the most likely diagnosis?

A Acne vulgaris
B Dermatomyositis
C Eczema
D Rosacea
E Systemic lupus erythematosus

42. Electrocardiogram (6)

You are covering the wards overnight. You are bleeped by the critical care ward. An experienced nurse informs you that a recent admission, an 83-year-old woman, has second-degree heart block. You ask her to fax the ECG to you as you are so busy.

What is meant by second-degree heart block?

A A bradycardic QRS complex is dissociated from the P-wave
B Occasional P-waves are failing to conduct through and trigger QRS complexes
C There is a prolonged P-R interval
D There is ST segment elevation throughout the chest leads
E The QRS complexes are irregularly irregular

43. Emergency management (2)

A 32-year-old man is brought to the emergency department whilst fitting. His airway has been secured using a Guedel airway. He has oxygen saturations above 96% on 15 L of oxygen and a capillary refill time of 2 seconds. Intravenous access has been gained.

Which of the following is the most appropriate next step?

A Jaw thrust
B Intravenous benzylpenicillin
C Intravenous lorazepam
D Intravenous phenytoin
E Rectal diazepam

44. Supraventricular tachycardia

A pleasantly confused 92-year-old woman with a history of cardiac disease is an inpatient on your ward. You are called by a nurse as her observations are peculiar and she is not feeling well. Her heart rate is 150 bpm and her blood pressure 110/60 mmHg. You inspect her electrocardiogram (ECG) and diagnose a supraventricular tachycardia.

A sensible next step would be to:

A Administer adenosine
B Administer digoxin
C Book an echocardiogram for tomorrow
D Defibrillate
E Print off the ECG and put it in the notes – no further action is required

45. Syndrome of inappropriate ADH secretion

A 68-year-old man presents to hospital with a 2-week history of confusion and he is found to have a pneumonia, for which he is treated. You note his plasma sodium is 119 mmol/L.

Which of the following investigation findings is consistent with a diagnosis of "syndrome of inappropriate anti-diuretic hormone secretion"?

(Normal values: urine osmolality 50–1200 mOsm/kg, plasma osmolality 280–300 mOsm/kg)

A Urine osmolality 45 mOsm/kg, plasma osmolality 250 mOsm/kg
B Urine osmolality 45 mOsm/kg, plasma osmolality 290 mOsm/kg
C Urine osmolality 45 mOsm/kg, plasma osmolality 305 mOsm/kg
D Urine osmolality 800 mOsm/kg, plasma osmolality 250 mOsm/kg
E Urine osmolality 800 mOsm/kg, plasma osmolality 305 mOsm/kg

46. Systemic lupus erythematosus (3)

A 26-year-old woman presents to the GP with right-sided pleuritic chest pain and increasing exertional dyspnoea that has lasted for about 2 weeks. She also complains of fatigue, malaise, hair loss and arthralgia that has lasted for 3 months. On examination, she has a rash over her cheeks, and auscultation of the chest reveals a friction rub and dullness to percussion over the right lower zone. Autoantibody blood tests demonstrate a profile consistent with systemic lupus erythematosus (SLE).

What is the most likely pulmonary manifestation of SLE in this case?

A Acute pleuritis
B Acute pneumonitis
C Interstitial lung disease
D Pneumonia
E Pulmonary haemorrhage

47. Urinary frequency (2)

A 48-year-old man presents to the emergency department in a reduced state of consciousness. He was brought in by his son who says he has been more confused over the past few days. A collateral history suggests 2 weeks of polyuria and polydipsia. There was no history of head injury, trauma or ingestion of illegal drugs. He has no other significant past medical history. He has a 21 unit/week alcohol history. On examination, he is unresponsive to pain. The liver edge is felt on abdominal examination. His blood tests show:

Na^+	168 mmol/L
K^+	3.8 mmol/L
Glucose	68 mmol/L
Serum osmolality	350 mmol/kg
Urea	14.3 mmol/L
Creatinine	203 µmol/L

A urine dipstick test revealed glycosuria but no ketones

What is the most likely differential diagnosis?

A Diabetic ketoacidosis
B Encephalitis
C Hepatic encephalopathy
D Hyperosmolar non-ketotic diabetic coma
E Uraemia

48. Wilson's disease

A 24-year-old man diagnosed with Wilson's disease was started on penicillamine. He calls his GP 1 month later to report that he has a temperature and a sore throat and has noticed marked bruising in the last week.

What advice should the GP give at this time?

A Advise the patient this is likely to be flu
B Ask the patient to come in for an urgent blood test
C Ask the patient to take some paracetamol and book an appointment the following week
D Increase the dose of penicillamine
E Reconsider the diagnosis of Wilson's disease

49. X-ray changes in osteoarthritis

Which of the following radiographic changes are NOT consistent with a diagnosis of osteoarthritis?

A Loss of joint space
B Osteophytes
C Punched-out periarticular erosions
D Subarticular sclerosis
E Subchondral cysts

50. Traveller's diarrhoea

A 22-year-old male medical student returns from travelling across Southeast Asia with a 48-hour history of watery diarrhoea and abdominal pain. He is otherwise well in himself.

What is the commonest organism for a short history of traveller's diarrhoea?

A Ameobic dysentery
B *Escherichia coli*
C *Listeria*
D Malaria
E *Salmonella*

Practice Paper 6: Answers

1. Amenorrhoea

B. Karyotype analysis

This patient has Turner's syndrome, characterised by short stature and primary amenorrhoea due to loss of part or all of an X chromosome. Other features include a broad square-shaped chest, widely spaced nipples, a webbed neck, a high palate and short fourth metacarpals. Most affected females have no pubertal development and primary amenorrhoea. There are some who develop normally and have secondary amenorrhoea. Patients with Turner's syndrome may have other complications such as renal anomalies, cardiovascular disease/abnormalities (coarctation of the aorta, aortic valvular disease, aortic dissection, hypertension), osteoporosis, ocular abnormalities and hypothyroidism. Karyotype analysis is used to analyse the chromosomal composition of the individual, which would reveal an abnormal or missing X chromosome in these females (45XO).

Henry Turner, American endocrinologist (1892-1970)

2. Myasthenia gravis

D. Rimmed vacuoles on muscle biopsy

In the tensilon test, edrophonium (a very short acting cholinesterase inhibitor) is administered and if positive, the weakness markedly improves for around 2–4 minutes. Positivity suggests myasthenia gravis although it can be positive in the Lambert–Eaton myasthenic syndrome. Electromyography commonly reveals that with repeated stimulation of the motor nerve fibres, the amplitude of the muscle action potentials reduce – a "decrementing response". This seems to represent the classic fatigability of the weakness in myasthenia gravis. A more sensitive test is looking at "jitter" – the variability of action potential time interval between two different single motor fibres of the same motor unit. Acetylcholine receptor antibodies are found in at least 90% of patients and, with increased sensitivity of new assays, it is thought that 96% actually may be positive. In many negative patients, antibodies to muscle-specific kinase (MuSK) are found. In any new patient, a CT of the chest should be carried out to look for thymoma, found in 10% of patients. Hyperplasia is found in a further 70% of patients. Rimmed vacuoles are in fact a hallmark of the rare inclusion body myositis. Muscle biopsy may reveal muscle fibre atrophy and can show small necrotic foci of damage or diffuse necrosis and inflammation, depending on disease severity.

3. Hyperkalaemia

B. Deepening Q-waves

A potassium level >7 mmol/L is a medical emergency and can be asymptomatic until arrest. ECG monitoring should be set up to look for early changes, and the ECG compared to a previous ECG from when the patient was stable (if available). The T-waves tent because potassium influx into cells drives repolarisation, and ventricular repolarisation is represented by the T-wave – the higher extracellular potassium concentrations lead to a larger magnitude of depolarisation. The P-waves flatten (although this may be subtle) and the QRS complexes broaden. Finding of any of these changes should increase urgency of treatment, during which ECG monitoring should continue. The changes progress to reveal a "sine wave" pattern, and ventricular fibrillation can ensue if appropriate treatment is not instituted. Deepening Q-waves would be associated with evolution of an ST-elevation myocardial infarction, with the initial ST elevation decreasing and the Q-waves deepening hours to days after the infarct.

4. Myocardial infarction

D. Nuclear studies of the myocardium

Single photon emission computerised tomography (SPECT) is a nuclear medicine scan involving gamma rays. It relies on the injection of a gamma-emitting radioisotope (a radionuclide), which is taken up by healthy myocardium. A sequence of images of the myocardium is then taken to highlight any perfusion deficiencies and ventricular dysfunction. Infarcted myocardium will be clearly displayed. Troponin tests can also be positive in heart failure and are therefore not sensitive enough in this context.

5. Pruritus

A. Electrolytes

A full blood count can reveal anaemia (which may be due to iron deficiency), polycythaemia, lymphoma or leukaemia, all of which can cause pruritus. Polycythaemia characteristically causes itching upon bathing. Iron studies can reveal a low ferritin and thus iron deficiency, which can cause pruritus. A cause should be sought (e.g. gastrointestinal bleeding, menorrhagia, diet). Hyperthyroidism and hypothyroidism can both cause itching. Chronic renal failure can cause an intractable pruritus, which unfortunately is often not relieved by dialysis, thus measuring urea is useful. Electrolyte abnormalities do not cause pruritus. A full and thorough history and examination can guide towards a potential diagnosis, however subclinical disease may be evident on blood tests, hence the pruritus screen. Other indicated blood tests include liver function tests (bile salt deposited in the skin can cause itching). If all is negative, psychological factors can often play a part, with anxiety being the most common cause. The tests can be repeated at intervals if patients re-present and/or psychological factors seem unlikely.

Pruritus, from Latin *prurire* = to itch

6. Seizures

C. Shooting/electric shock-like pains in the limbs

Complex partial seizures usually originate in the temporal lobe, and can affect various components of the limbic system (including the hippocampus). The limbic system has various functions including memory, emotion, taste and smell, and consciousness. Therefore, complex partial seizures present with episodes of clouding of consciousness combined with various symptoms that may include visceral symptoms (fullness, choking, nausea, tachycardia, taste and smell hallucinations), memory disturbance (déjà-vu, jamais-vu, derealisation, flashbacks, formed auditory or visual hallucinations), motor disturbances of a semi-purposeful nature, or intense paroxysmal mood disturbance. Shooting pains into the limbs, depending on the distribution, sounds typical of a radiculopathy, and "electric-shock" sensations sounds like "Lhermitte's sign", a sign in multiple sclerosis with cervical posterior column involvement, whereby sudden neck flexion causes electric-shock sensations in the limbs. Focal somatosensory or pain information is not processed in the temporal lobe or limbic system anyhow, so is unlikely to be caused by complex partial seizures.

Jean Lhermitte, French neurologist (1877-1959)

7. Spinal cord compression

D. T10

Complete involvement of the legs, in either sensory or motor modality indicates that the lesion is higher than L1. The arms are normal, so the lesion is lower than T1. Getting the answer then depends on knowledge of anatomical landmarks of spinal sensory levels. T_4 is the level of the nipples, which does not help us narrow the answer down. T10 is the level of the bellybutton, and thus T10 is the answer we are looking for. The cause of greatest concern is metastases – magnetic resonance imaging (MRI) of the spine may discover this or another cause, and gauge the extent of spinal compression if that is indeed the cause.

8. Sepsis

C. Neutrophils < 0.5 × 10⁹/L

The combination of a raised temperature and low neutrophils (<1 or <0.5 × 10^9/L according to local policy) is described as neutropenic sepsis. Patients receiving chemotherapy often drop their neutrophil count due to bone marrow suppression, and the relative paucity of neutrophils means that the host defence against bacteria is severely compromised. These patients can die rapidly despite not being clinically drastically unwell. It is essential to start broad-spectrum intravenous antibiotics as soon as possible. Blood cultures can be taken afterwards if necessary.

9. Radiographic changes in ankylosing spondylitis

D. Sacroiliitis

Fusion of the sacroiliac joints and fusion of the lumbar vertebra (giving the "bamboo spine") happen only after prolonged persistent inflammation leads to calcification of the ligaments. Osteophytes are seen in osteoarthritis and in degenerative spinal disease (spondylosis). Syndesmophytes are bony spurs caused by persistent inflammation that are more vertically oriented than osteophytes and represent an earlier stage of disease than bamboo spine. The earliest radiographic change in ankylosing spondylitis is sacroiliitis.

10. Management of toxicity

D. Give intravenous naloxone

Opiate toxicity in patients causes reduced consciousness, respiratory depression, pinpoint pupils and hypotension. In the case of reduced conscious level or respiratory depression, aliquots of 0.4 mg to 2.0 mg intravenous naloxone should be given and the dose might need repeating if there is inadequate response after 2 minutes. A naloxone infusion might be needed in the case of known severe opiate toxicity (e.g. long-acting opiates such as MST or methadone). N-acetylcysteine is used in paracetamol overdose. Flumazenil is used in benzodiazepine overdose. Sodium bicarbonate is used in salicylate poisoning. Torsades de pointes induced by anti-depressant overdose (e.g. selective serotonin reuptake inhibitors) is treated with intravenous magnesium sulphate.

11. Squamous cell carcinoma

A. Curettage is the first line of management

Curettage is unlikely to remove the whole tumour and will lead to delay in clearance of the malignant cells. Primary excision should be the first line of management. Mohs micrographic surgery, whereby excised samples are examined under the microscope at the time of excision, and then further tissue resected until the margins are clear, can be used for high-risk recurrent lesions. Radiotherapy can be used where excision is not possible, and chemotherapy can be used in metastatic disease. Sun exposure is indeed a risk factor for squamous cell carcinoma, which tends to be ill-defined keratotic ulcerating lesions. They are more common in kidney transplant patients because of the long-term immunosuppression – another risk factor. Unlike basal cell carcinomas, squamous cell carcinomas can indeed metastasise, usually to lymph nodes, so if histopathology confirms a squamous cell carcinoma, annual follow-up for 5 years to exclude lymphadenopathy or recurrent malignancy is recommended.

Frederic Edward Mohs, American surgeon (1910-2002)

12. Management of urinary tract infection

A. All of the results below require treatment

Presence of either leukocyte esterase or nitrites makes a urinary tract infection likely, as both are specific tests. Absence of both makes a urinary tract infection unlikely, however in pregnancy the risk of ascending infection and renal damage is higher and any evidence of bacteriuria warrants antibiotic treatment and further investigation, e.g. by ultrasound.

13. Side effects of anti-tuberculous medication

A. Ethambutol

Ethambutol can cause optic neuritis, which initially affects the myelinated nerves supplying the cones in the fovea. Thus, loss of colour vision and visual acuity can be the earliest presenting features. If picked up early, stopping the ethambutol can lead to reversal of the process and the vision saved. Isoniazid, pyrazinamide and rifampicin along with the ethambutol comprise standard quadruple therapy, which will be given for the first 2 months in new tuberculosis, before continuing the isoniazid and rifampicin for a further 4 months. All three can cause hepatitis. Isoniazid can cause peripheral neuropathy via a vitamin B_6 deficiency, so prophylactic pyridoxine is prescribed. Rifampicin is an enzyme inducer and can interact with many other medications, notably the oral contraceptive pill. It can also turn body secretions orange. Streptomycin can be used in place of ethambutol or in combination with all four in resistant tuberculosis.

14. Hypothyroidism

A. Amiodarone

Amiodarone has a chemical structure that is analogous to thyroxine and contains large amounts of iodine. Amiodarone has a cytotoxic effect on thyroid follicular cells and inhibits conversion of T_4 to T_3. As a result, either hypothyroidism (Wolff–Chaikoff effect) or hyperthyroidism (Jod–Basedow effect) may occur. Thyroid function tests should be done before commencement of amiodarone and thyroid-stimulating hormone should be measured every 6 months whilst the patient is on treatment.

15. Painful fingers

B. Limited cutaneous systemic sclerosis

Systemic sclerosis is a connective tissue disorder characterised by thickening and fibrosis of the skin (scleroderma) with involvement of internal organs. There are two forms: 1) a limited cutaneous type (60%) and 2) a diffuse cutaneous type (40%). Limited cutaneous scleroderma is limited to the distal limbs (i.e. distal to the elbows and knees). Other features include a beaked nose and small, furrowed mouth (microstoma). Limited cutaneous scleroderma also encompasses CREST syndrome, which is characterised by Calcinosis, Raynaud phenomenon, oEsophageal dysmotility, Sclerodactyly and Telangiectasia. Calcinosis is the formation of calcium deposits in the soft tissues, often seen on the pulps of the fingers. Raynaud phenomenon is an idiopathic condition with episodic digital vasospasm precipitated by a cold environment, as a result of which the affected fingers or toes become white and may be painful. Oesophageal dysmotility is manifest as dysphagia and reflux. Sclerodactyly describes the presence of tight, shiny skin over the fingers, producing a fixed flexion deformity. In limited cutaneous scleroderma the anti-centromere antibody is characteristically positive. Pulmonary hypertension is a common internal manifestation.

Diffuse cutaneous scleroderma can involve the whole skin of the body. Patients are characteristically positive for the anti-SCL-70 antibody (also known as anti-topoisomerase II). In this form of disease, patients are particularly at risk of a 'renal crisis' – a life-threatening malignant hypertension with rapid renal impairment. By contrast, pulmonary hypertension is less common. Diffuse cutaneous systemic sclerosis has a worse prognosis than limited cutaneous disease. The treatment of systemic sclerosis is with steroids and immunosuppressives. Penicillamine slows skin disease (steroids do not help the skin). Lung fibrosis is the main cause of death, followed by renal disease.

Scleroderma can occur without internal organ disease (localised scleroderma). If this occurs in plaques it is known as morphea; if it occurs in lines it is termed *en coup de sabre*. "Scleroderma *sine* scleroderma" is the name given for patients who have typical vascular or internal organ features of systemic sclerosis but without the cutaneous sclerosis.

Dermatomyositis, another connective tissue disease, can feature dilated nail-fold capillary loops, but this presentation is not of dermatomyositis – we would expect a proximal muscle weakness and pain with possible skin manifestations including heliotropic rash around the eyes and Gottron's papules on the dorsum of the hands.

Morphea, from Greek *morpha* = shape

En coup de sabre, from French = cut of the sword

Scleroderma, from Latin *skleros* = hard + *dermis* = skin

Maurice Raynaud, French physician (1834-1881)

16. Palpitations (3)

A. 24-hour electrocardiogram

The clinical features of this patient suggest thyrotoxicosis. Patients with primary thyrotoxicosis would have raised T_3 and T_4 with an undetectable TSH. TSH receptor antibody levels are raised in Graves disease. An ECG may demonstrate atrial fibrillation. The Technetium-99 scintigraphy scan would demonstrate the distribution of the uptake of the isotope: 1) in Graves disease there is a diffuse uptake of isotope, 2) in multinodular goitre there is low patchy uptake within the nodules, and 3) in toxic adenomas there is lack of uptake of isotope by the normal dormant gland. Fine-needle aspiration confirms the cytology of the thyroid nodule. A 24-hour electrocardiogram (ECG) may demonstrate atrial fibrillation but it is not essential in the diagnosis of thyrotoxicosis.

17. Haemoptysis (2)

B. Idiopathic pulmonary haemosiderosis

Idiopathic pulmonary haemosiderosis is a rare condition with unknown aetiology that is characterised by recurrent episodes of alveolar haemorrhage and haemoptysis (in the absence of renal disease) and leads to iron deficiency anaemia. Most patients present in childhood with 85% of cases having an onset of symptoms before 16 years of age. The aetiology is thought to be multifactorial with possible associations with toxin exposure and an autoimmune mechanism. The alveolar and interstitial spaces are filled with haemosiderin-laden macrophages with variable extent of interstitial fibrosis and degeneration of alveolar, interstitial and vascular elastic fibres. The clinical course of this condition ranges from continuous low-level bleeding to massive pulmonary haemorrhage. Continuous pulmonary haemorrhage leads to the chronic non-productive cough with haemoptysis, malaise, lethargy and failure to thrive in children. Chronic bleeding leads to iron deficiency anaemia, chronic disabling dyspnoea, pulmonary fibrosis and cor pulmonale.

18. Antibody testing

B. Anti-glomerular basement membrane antibodies (anti-GBM)

This patient has Goodpasture's syndrome, which is a rare condition in which autoantibodies are formed against the glomerular basement membrane and the alveolar membrane. The antibodies trigger a type 2 hypersensitivity reaction that causes renal failure, pulmonary haemorrhage and haemoptysis. The condition is usually diagnosed by the detection of anti-GBM in the serum and via renal biopsy. The biopsy often shows focal or diffuse crescentic glomerulonephritis. Immunofluorescence may demonstrate linear deposition of IgG antibodies and complement (C3) on the glomerular basement membrane. Goodpasture's syndrome is usually treated aggressively with plasmapheresis, corticosteroids and immunosuppression.

Anti-dsDNA antibodies are found in systemic lupus erythematosis, and whilst only 60% are sensitive (compared to >95% with ANA), it is far more specific. Lupus can cause renal disease, typically with proteinuria and/or casts rather than haematuria, and can affect the lungs through pleuritis or pleural effusions but it does not cause haemoptysis. Anti-ribonucleoprotein antibodies are specific for mixed connective tissue disease, which would be unlikely to give the present clinical picture. Cytoplasmic anti-neutrophil cytoplasm antibodies (cANCA) are most associated with Wegener's granulomatosis, which could cause a similar picture with renal impairment of a nephritic type and haemoptysis. It is also sometimes found in Churg–Strauss syndrome, microscopic polyangiitis, and polyarteritis nodosa. Perinuclear anti-neutrophil cytoplasmic antibodies (pANCA) are found most often in microscopic polyangiitis, and can actually sometimes be positive in Goodpasture's syndrome.

Ernest William Goodpasture, American pathologist (1886-1960)

19. Management of shortness of breath (4)

A. Consider intravenous dexamethasone and radiotherapy

Superior vena cava syndrome is a clinical condition that occurs due to obstruction of the superior vena cava. The most common aetiology is malignancy (65% of cases) and is followed by benign causes, which include iatrogenic causes (e.g. central venous catheters, pacemaker), mediastinal fibrosis caused by radiotherapy or infections, collagen-vascular diseases (e.g. sarcoidosis or Behçet syndrome), and rarely, mediastinal haematoma, substernal goitre and aortic arch aneurysm. The most common malignant cause is lung cancer, followed by lymphoma, metastatic breast cancer and metastatic colon cancer. Patients present with dyspnoea, cough, facial plethora and oedema, oedema of the upper extremities, distended neck veins and chest veins and, in severe cases, they have stridor related to laryngeal oedema or direct compression. Oxygen should be provided to correct hypoxaemia. A chest X-ray might reveal a widened mediastinum and a mass lesion. Airway management is important as the patient might have upper airway obstruction due to severe oedema and intubation should be considered in these cases. Corticosteroids and radiation therapy or percutaneous stenting are considered for the relief of obstructive symptoms. Urgent combination therapy with radiotherapy and corticosteroids are only used in life-threatening situations as they might cause interference with subsequent histopathological diagnosis in patients who do not have histopathological evidence of malignancy.

20. Atrial fibrillation

A. Abdominal aortic aneurysm

Atrial fibrillation commonly presents with either missing P-waves on the electrocardiogram (ECG), or, as beautifully described in 1876 by Carl Nothnagel:

> "In this form of arrhythmia the heartbeats follow each other in complete irregularity. At the same time, the height and tension of the individual pulse waves are continuously changing".

Because the atria are not efficiently contracting, blood can clot within the left atrium and result in embolisation.

Causes of atrial fibrillation can be remembered using 'Dehydrated PIRATES':

- Dehydration
- Pulmonary disease, e.g. pulmonary embolism
- Ischaemia (hypertension, ischaemic heart disease, heart failure)
- Rheumatic heart disease
- Anaemia, atrial myxoma
- Thyrotoxicosis
- Ethanol abuse
- Sepsis

21. Blood groups

C. AB+

Blood groups A and B represent antigens present on the surface of the red blood cell. Blood type O indicates the absence of these antigens. Through our diets we are exposed to all antigens and therefore build up antibodies to any foreign antigens, for example a person with blood type O, and therefore no native antigen chains (universal donor if Rhesus negative), will have antibodies to both A and B chains. However, a person who has both AB on their own cells will not produce antibodies and can therefore receive all blood (universal recipient if Rhesus positive). Although the ABO compatibility is the most important blood typing system, more than 30 other blood typing systems are known. Rhesus compatibility is demonstrated by the plus or minus symbol.

22. Generalised weakness

B. Cushing's syndrome

Cushing's syndrome is caused by the excessive activation of glucocorticoid receptors. The most common cause of Cushing's syndrome is iatrogenic secondary to prolonged use of synthetic glucocorticoids such as prednisolone. The degree to which symptoms manifest is dependent on the degree of cortisol excess. Patients will complain of abnormal weight gain, acne, striae, abnormal bruising and weakness involving their proximal muscles. They may be found to be hyperglycaemic, hypertensive and are prone to infections with poor wound healing. A history of poor asthma control suggests that patient is on long-term steroid therapy, which is the main cause of her Cushing's syndrome.

Harvey Williams Cushing, American neurosurgeon (1869-1939)

23. Investigation of jaundice

E. Paracetamol levels

This patient is most likely to have taken an overdose of paracetamol, which has resulted in the features of acute liver failure demonstrated above. Alcohol can cause a similar picture in the long term but not in the acute setting. Paracetamol overdose in the first 24 hours presents with non-specific symptoms of nausea and vomiting. Hepatic necrosis begins 24 hours after the overdose with the classical signs of acute liver failure. Initial investigations need to include liver function tests (LFTs), paracetamol and salicylate levels, blood glucose (as such patients are prone to hypoglycaemia), urea and electrolytes (think hepatorenal syndrome, although urea is synthesised in the liver and so may not be deranged), clotting and an arterial blood gas looking for lactic acidosis. If patients with a paracetamol overdose present within 1 hour you can consider giving activated charcoal to prevent absorption. A 4-hour paracetamol level can be used to determine which patients would benefit from N-acetylcysteine infusions. Maximum protection is gained by giving the antidote within 8 hours of ingestion.

24. Management of skin conditions

A. All clothes, bedsheets and any upholstery contacted by the patient should be washed thoroughly

Scabies is caused by parasitic mites that burrow under the skin and lay their eggs, eventually causing a hypersensitivity reaction that causes the itch. Washing underwear and nightclothes suffices to cover potential lurking mites that may re-infect the individual after treatment. Burrows, which can often be linear lesions representing the path burrowed by the mite, have a vesicle at the end of the mite, and are indeed often found in the web spaces of fingers and toes, as well as hands and feet, wrists and ankles, elbows, nipples and male genitalia. For diagnosis, a burrow (not those on the genitalia) should be scraped off and examined under the microscope directly. A dermatoscope can sometimes visualise the mite *in situ* in the burrow on the patient. Malathion and permethrin are both valid topical treatments, which should be applied all over. Permethrin can be washed off after 12 hours, malathion after 24 hours. A second application 7 days later is often recommended to sweep up any mites missed by the first treatment.

Scabies, from Latin *scabere* = to itch

25. Investigation of muscle weakness

B. Multifocal decreased motor conduction speed with/without conduction block

Guillain–Barré syndrome (GBS) is the eponym for acute inflammatory postinfectious polyneuropathy. It commonly follows viral infection, e.g. varicella zoster virus, mumps, cytomegalovirus, or bacterial infections such as *Campylobacter* or *Mycoplasma*. However, serology confirming prior infection with one of these organisms does not confirm GBS. Lumbar puncture commonly reveals raised protein, but lymphocytes are not usually raised and oligoclonal bands would not be expected. The underlying pathology is an autoimmune attack on the myelin in the peripheral nerves, and so slowed motor conduction speed would be expected. If the inflammation is severe then axons can be damaged, giving a conduction block picture. This indicates that a degree of irreversible damage has taken place. There is a 2% mortality rate in GBS, and of those who develop respiratory failure, 20% are left severely disabled. Therapy is with intravenous immunoglobulin if the patient is unable to walk.

Georges Guillain, French neurologist (1876-1961)

Jean Alexandre Barré, French neurologist (1880-1967)

26. Hepatitis serology

A. Acute hepatitis B infection

The immunological tests for hepatitis B can be complicated and confusing, however they can be very helpful in determining the current hepatitis status of the patient as well as their previous exposure. Hepatitis B is a DNA virus that is mainly transmitted via blood products and sexual activity. Certain individuals, such as those who work in healthcare, are required to be vaccinated against hepatitis B. The vaccine contains the hepatitis surface antigen (HBsAg) against which the immune system produces hepatitis B surface antibody (HBsAb). It is HBsAb that is measured after vaccination to evaluate the response to the vaccine. Some individuals have a poor response to the vaccine and require higher doses of vaccine or booster shots. HBsAb are also found in patients who have had hepatitis in the past. In this situation the patient will also have developed antibodies to the hepatitis B core antigen (HBcAg), which is not present in patients who have been immunised.

Hepatitis B surface antigen (HBsAg) can usually be detected within 4 weeks of infection and is the earliest marker of hepatitis B infection. It is not found in patients vaccinated against hepatitis B. If HBsAg is still detected in the serum 6 months after an acute hepatitis B infection, the patient has become a chronic carrier of the virus. The risk of developing chronic hepatitis B infection is related to age at the time of infection. The majority of infected neonates develop chronic infection whereas only 5–10% of adults do so.

Hepatitis B e antigen (HBeAg) can be present in both acute and chronic hepatitis B and indicates a high level of infectivity. The presence of HBeAg in chronic hepatitis B suggests that the patient is infective and has an aggressive disease requiring treatment. In addition to establishing infectivity, the measurement of HBeAg can be used to assess the efficacy of treatment with falling levels indicating success. It should be noted that there are some mutant strains of the hepatitis B virus found in Asia and the Middle East that do not produce HBeAg. Hepatitis B DNA levels can also be used to assess disease activity with high levels indicating active disease and infectivity.

Hepatitis B core antibodies (HBcAb) can be present in acute and chronic infection. They are formed against the hepatitis B core antigen (HBcAg), which is found within the liver and therefore cannot be detected using serology. In acute infection it is the second marker to be detected, after HBsAb, and is usually seen after 4 weeks of infection. In chronic disease the presence of high titres of HBcAb, in the absence of HBeAg, indicates low infectivity and disease activity. This serological picture is associated with a better prognosis with fewer individuals progressing to cirrhosis and hepatocellular carcinoma.

27. Lumbar puncture

D. Tubercular meningitis

The glucose is low, indicating excessive glucose consumption, which rules out viral meningitis. The predominance of lymphocytes suggests a more chronic infection and rules out bacterial meningitis. The negative India ink stain rules out cryptococcal meningitis. Finally, the extremely large number of lymphocytes and amount of protein make tuberculosis more likely than malignant meningitis. Ziehl–Neelsen staining or PCR would confirm the diagnosis. However, clinical information, conspicuously absent from this case, would be extremely useful.

28. Management of hyperkalaemia

A. Calcium gluconate

Hyperkalaemia is defined as a serum potassium level of >5 mmol/L, but severe hyperkalaemia, with a serum potassium level of >7 mmol/L, is a medical emergency. ECG monitoring should be instituted and intravenous access sought. Calcium gluconate does not lower serum potassium, but 10 ml of 10% calcium gluconate is given as a cardioprotective agent as it is a cardiac membrane stabiliser and protects against cardiac arrhythmias. This should be given soon as it can buy time to lower the potassium level. Dextrose (50 ml of 50% solution) with 10 U Actrapid insulin can be given intravenously – insulin drives potassium rapidly into cells and the dextrose is given with it to avoid hypoglycaemia. Potassium and glucose levels should then be monitored repeatedly. Calcium resonium, typically given as a 30 mg suppository, soaks up potassium from the bowel wall, and then an enema after 9 hours will actually remove potassium from the body. Calcium resonium can also be given orally (15 mg t.d.s.) with laxatives to speed transit time. The cause for the high potassium should be sought and reversed where possible. Medications such as beta-blockers, angiotensin-converting enzyme (ACE) inhibitors, potassium-sparing diuretics such as spironolactone, and NSAIDs can contribute and should be stopped. Hyperglycaemia can be responsible, as can causes of cell lysis such as burns and rhabdomyolysis. Acute or chronic renal failure are often responsible, and if acute renal failure is not reversible by other means then dialysis will be needed and this often is the definitive means of reducing the serum potassium. Furosemide is a loop diuretic and causes potassium loss through the kidney but if the patient is clinically dry or has renal failure this may be unsafe. Salbutamol nebulisers can be used to drive potassium into cells, but the high doses needed lead to side effects such as tachycardia, anxiety and tremors, which are undesirable in an already unwell patient.

29. Management of hypertension

A. ACE inhibitors

Diabetic nephropathy is among the most common causes of end-stage renal failure in developed countries. Microalbuminuria is an important indicator of risk of developing overt diabetic nephropathy. Blood pressure control is associated with reduction of proteinuria, and a reduction in the rate of chronic kidney disease progression. Angiotensin-converting enzyme (ACE) inhibitors dilate the efferent renal arteriole, thus reducing intraglomerular hypertension and proteinuria, regardless of whether blood pressure is elevated or not.

30. Malabsorption

A. Exclusion of gluten from the diet

Coeliac disease causes a gluten-related enteropathy of the small bowel. When the patient consumes gluten-containing foods, a T-cell mediated autoimmune reaction results in subtotal villous atrophy and crypt hyperplasia of the small bowel mucosa. Specifically, it is gliadin – a constituent of gluten – which causes the immunological response. The result is malabsorption leading to malnutrition, anaemia, steatorrhoea, abdominal pain, bloating and fatigue. The initial investigation for coeliac disease is the measurement of serum anti-endomyseal or anti-transglutaminase IgA antibodies, which have been shown to have sensitivities and specificities of over 95%. Antibodies to alpha-gliadin and reticulin can also be measured although they have lower sensitivities and specificities. The gold standard diagnostic technique is duodenal or jejunal biopsy taken during endoscopy. Gluten exclusion can reverse the disease process, and therefore biopsy must occur before exclusion starts. Since this is an invasive and unpleasant procedure it is usually performed as a second-line investigation in patients with positive serology. If the biopsy suggests coeliac disease the patient should be placed on a gluten-free diet and re-biopsied at a later date to assess small bowel recovery.

31. Brain tumours

D. A 50-year-old woman with insidious onset unilateral deafness, on Weber's testing sound is louder contralaterally, and with some ipsilateral reduced facial sensation

The 65-year-old man most likely has presbyacusis – reduced ability to hear high-frequency sounds with ageing. The 40-year-old woman with insidious unilateral deafness experiences sound louder on the affected side with Weber's testing – this is indicative of conductive rather than sensorineural deafness. There is also no other neurology mentioned. Regarding cerebellopontine angle tumours, the most common is the vestibular schwannoma (formerly known as the misleading "acoustic neuroma"), representing 80% thereof. The café au lait spots of the 30-year-old woman are indicative of neurofibromatosis type 1 (von Recklinghausen disease). This neurocutaneous syndrome is not in fact associated with vestibular schwannomas – whereas neurofibromatosis type 2 is. This syndrome typically presents with bilateral vestibular schwannomas, and rarely are café au lait spots a feature. Furthermore, facial weakness coming on over days with no other neurological deficit is not typical of a cerebellopontine angle lesion. Cranial nerves V, VII and VIII are typically involved in a cerebellopontine angle lesion – although facial weakness can often be absent despite marked compression. The man with bilateral facial weakness, nasal voice and swallowing difficulty appears to have widespread involvement of the lower motor cranial nerves – a bulbar palsy – his age and the speed of onset should raise suspicion of motor neuron disease. That leaves the 50-year-old woman with sensorineural deafness of insidious onset (Weber's louder contralaterally) and some reduced ipsilateral facial numbness (V nerve involvement). The unilateral sensorineural deafness of slow onset is typical and is due to the slow-growing benign tumour compressing the VIII nerve. Vertigo is uncommon as compensatory mechanisms can act over the long time period. If the tumour grows larger than 2 cm in diameter, the V nerve can be compressed giving pain, numbness and paraesthesia. Cerebellar symptoms may appear with very large tumours, and rarely fourth ventricle compression can give a raised intracranial pressure.

32. Chest injury

A. Beck's triad

Beck's triad of muffled heart sounds, engorged neck veins and hypotension indicate acute cardiac tamponade, in this case caused by a stab wound to the myocardium. The resultant haemorrhage fills the fibrous pericardium, reducing the space available for the heart to fill in systole. Diastolic volume is therefore steadily reduced as the haemorrhage continues, leading to a possibly fatal reduction in cardiac output. Pericardiocentesis is required acutely: a cannula is inserted to the left of the xiphisternum under cardiac monitoring (an electrocardiogram (ECG) change can indicate contact with the myocardium, i.e. that you've gone too far). Upon penetrating the pericardium, the blood can be drained and cardiac output restored. Beck also performed the first defribrillation in 1947 with equipment made to his design, by his friend James Rand Jr, who also invented the electric shaver (under the Remington brand).

Kussmaul's sign is a raised jugular venous pressure (JVP) upon inspiration that falls in expiration and is seen in constrictive pericarditis. This does not happen reliably in acute cardiac tamponade, where neck veins remain distended throughout respiration. Kussmaul also first described the deep, slow and laboured breathing pattern that occurs late in the severe metabolic acidosis of diabetic ketoacidosis and renal failure.

A Stokes–Adams attack is syncope, with or without seizures, resulting from a transiently reduced cardiac output and can occur in any position and during sleep. Virchow's triad describes the thrombotic risk factors of hypercoagulability, venous stasis and endothelial injury.

Claude Beck, American cardiac surgeon (1894-1971)

Adolph Kussmaul, German physician (1822-1902)

33. Complications of hepatitis infection

C. Hepatocellular carcinoma

Chronic hepatitis B and C infections are associated with a significantly increased risk of hepatocellular carcinoma. Hepatocellular carcinoma is also an important consequence of liver cirrhosis and should be suspected in any patient with rapid development of weight loss on a background of cirrhosis. Within the general population the prevalence is four per 100 000 people. Investigations include serum alpha-fetoprotein, followed by either liver biopsy or computed tomography (CT) imaging. Resection is possible for early-stage cancers. The prognosis is extremely poor for non-resectable tumours, and there is a 20% 5-year survival rate for operable tumours.

34. Conn's syndrome

C. Conn's syndrome causes excess aldosterone, the vasoconstriction from which leads to hypertension

Primary hyperaldosteronism is a cause of excess aldosterone secretion, which leads to increased serum sodium concentration irrespective of plasma renin concentration. It is named Conn's syndrome if this is due to an aldosterone-secreting adrenal adenoma. This is the cause in <5% of cases; 70% are caused by bilateral idiopathic adrenal hyperplasia. The increased plasma sodium causes fluid retention, which leads to hypertension. Aldosterone is secreted by the adrenal glands and stimulates the kidneys to retain sodium (and excrete more potassium). The diuretic spironolactone is an aldosterone antagonist that will retain potassium and shed sodium and hence cause diuresis. Loop diuretics like furosemide and bumetanide cause a much more profound diuresis by inhibiting sodium/potassium/chloride reabsorption and hence potassium is lost.

35. Dysphagia

E. Oesophageal carcinoma

The man has several risk factors and warning signs for carcinoma: significant weight loss, smoking history of many packs a year and a dysphagia for solids. All these factors warrant an urgent 2-week referral for oesophageal carcinoma and endoscopic evaluation. Oesophageal carcinoma may be adenocarcinoma or squamous, with the trend to increasing numbers of adenocarcinomas over the traditional squamous. Histology also varies with location in the oesophagus. The major risk factors for oesophageal carcinoma include smoking and alcohol intake, as well as the presence of Barrett's oesophagus in adenocarcinoma. Epstein–Barr virus infection has also been linked to the aetiology of the disease. Oesophageal carcinoma often presents late in the course of the illness and hence holds a relatively poor prognosis. Treatment may be with radical surgery, radiotherapy or palliative stenting. The 5-year survival rate for resectable tumours is 10–25%.

36. Diagnosis of chest infection (2)

C. *Legionella* spp.

This patient has severe community-acquired pneumonia (she is confused, urea is raised, and she is aged >65). *Legionella* species can cause a severe bilateral pneumonia in middle to old age. It can be associated with local epidemics originating in cooling towers or water reservoirs. It is a Gram-negative aerobic bacterium. Urinary antigen testing can quickly diagnose and thus guide antibiotic therapy. *Escherichia coli* is more commonly causative of hospital-acquired pneumonia. An antigen test for viral causes of pneumonia would be clinically useless. *Mycoplasma pneumoniae* is more common in children and young adults.

Legionnaires' disease is so-called as it was first recognised as causing an outbreak of pneumonia in a group of elderly men attending an American Legion (war veteran) conference in Philadelphia

37. Diagnosis of cough (8)

A. Asthma

Asthma is characterised by chronic airway inflammation and increased airway hyper-responsiveness leading to symptoms of wheeze, cough, chest tightness and dyspnoea. The features that increase the probability of asthma include:

1. More than one of the following symptoms: wheeze, cough, breathlessness and chest tightness – particularly if symptoms are worse at night and in the early morning; if symptoms occur in response to exercise, allergen exposure and cold air; or if symptoms occur after taking aspirin and beta-blockers.
2. History of atopic disorder
3. Family history of asthma and/or atopic disorder
4. Widespread wheeze on auscultation
5. Otherwise unexplained low FEV_1 or PEF (historical or serial readings)
6. Otherwise unexplained peripheral blood eosinophilia

A diagnosis of asthma is made by compatible clinical history with either/ or:

1. FEV_1 ≥15% (and 200 ml) increase following administration of a bronchodilator/trial of corticosteroids
2. > 20% diurnal variation on ≥ 3 days in a week for 2 weeks on PEF diary
3. FEV_1 ≥15% decrease after 6 minutes of exercise.

Scottish Intercollegiate Guidelines Network (SIGN). British Guideline of the Management of Asthma. London: The British Thoracic Society 2008

38. Diagnosis of Cushing's syndrome

B. Computed tomography (CT) of the adrenals

The history suggests that this patient has ACTH-dependent Cushing's syndrome. Compared to ACTH-secreting pituitary tumours, ACTH-secreting ectopic tumours do not have residual negative feedback sensitivity to cortisol. Ectopic ACTH-secreting tumour is associated with very high ACTH and cortisol levels. A high ACTH level is associated with marked skin pigmentation, which is described by the patient as "tanned". A high cortisol level could cause profound hypokalaemia, severe muscle wasting and severe hyperglycaemia. An overnight low-dose dexamethasone suppression test, 48-hour high-dose dexamethasone suppression test and plasma ACTH test are used in the work-up of the diagnosis of ACTH-dependent Cushing's syndrome. Computed tomography (CT) of the chest is useful in detecting a possible bronchial origin of an ACTH-secreting tumour.

39. Diagnosis of neurological dysfunction (4)

C. Motor neurone disease

The lack of cerebellar involvement, optic neuritis, eye movement disorder, lack of sensory involvement and the patient's age all go against a diagnosis of multiple sclerosis (MS). In older patients MS is more likely to be primary progressive so the lack of relapses does not go against it necessarily. The patient seems to have a mixture of upper and lower motor neuron weakness in the limbs, which could go with cervical spondylosis, syringomyelia or motor neurone disease (MND) or MND-like syndromes. However the lack of sensory involvement points to MND or an MND-like syndrome. Syringomyelia starts with the lack of pain sensation in the arms before giving more prominent lower motor neuron weakness in the arms, and then later upper motor neuron weakness in the legs. Cervical spondylosis commonly presents with shooting pains into a dermatomal distribution in the arms, and would give upper motor neuron but not lower motor neuron signs in the legs. Brisk reflexes in a wasted limb is classic for MND, and comes from a combination of upper and lower motor neuron loss with an intact sensory input into the reflex loop. The patient's age is classic (>50), and progression swift, with patients typically dying 3–5 years from onset. Retroviruses such as HIV and polio (on a more limited scale, both in terms of affected limbs and worldwide disease burden with the introduction of improved sanitation and vaccines) can give lower and upper motor neuron loss with sparing of sensory neurons, and thus HIV can give an MND-like syndrome, however this patient does not have a travel history or medical history to make us consider this.

40. Diagnosis of rheumatoid arthritis (2)

B. Anti-CCP antibodies

ANCA is an antibody associated with small vessel vasculitides such as Wegener's granulomatosis and Churg–Strauss syndrome. Anti-centromere antibodies are associated with limited cutaneous systemic sclerosis. Rheumatoid factor is the traditional screening test for rheumatoid arthritis, however it is only positive in 70–80% of cases and it is present in many other autoimmune diseases, i.e. it lacks specificity. It is also present in 25% of the over-65s who do not have rheumatoid arthritis. Soft tissue swelling may be seen on X-ray of the hands but this is non-specific, and bony erosions are a late change that would not be expected in this case. Anti-cyclic citrullinated peptide (anti-CCP) antibody testing is 98% sensitive and far more specific to rheumatoid arthritis, and therefore represents a superior test. However it is important that diagnosis is made using the ACR criteria using clinical findings in addition to antibody tests.

41. Diagnosis of skin lesions (3)

D. Rosacea

The distribution (cheeks, nose) may be described as "malar" and the areas are all exposed to the sunlight. This makes a rash worsened by sunlight more likely. Whilst it is a typical distribution for the rash of systemic lupus erythematosus, this is a fairly rare condition. It also does not usually present with papules and pustules. Dermatomyositis is an extremely rare condition that can feature a heliotropic or sun-sensitive rash, as well as Gottron's papules on the hand and linear erythema on the dorsum of the hand, along with an inflammatory myositis. The qualities of the rash described above do not sound like eczema, which is typically dry and itchy and does not feature papules or pustules. Acne vulgaris does feature papules and pustules, usually on the face as well as the upper back and shoulders, but this typically affects those in the throes of puberty. Rosacea affects those in middle age, more typically women, and is more common than systemic lupus erythematosus, and does feature papules and pustules on a background of erythematous skin. The first-line treatment is oral tetracyclines (such as lymecycline).

Malar, from Latin *mala* = cheek-bone

Rosacea, from Latin *rosacea* = rose-coloured

42. Electrocardiogram (6)

B. Occasional P-waves are failing to conduct through and trigger QRS complexes

First-degree heart block is a prolonged P-R interval (>0.2 seconds). The P-wave is suffering a constant delay as it passes via the atrial-ventricular node (AVN). Second-degree heart block comes in two forms: either a P-R delay that increases with time until a beat is missed (Mobitz type 1 or Wenckebach block) or beats are missed in a ratio, i.e. every third beat (Mobitz type 2). Second-degree block is more serious and is best treated with pacing. Complete heart block (third degree) is more serious again. Beats are driven by a pacing focus distal to the AVN (normally at a bradycardic pace) and the P-wave is therefore dissociated from the QRS complexes. These patients are vulnerable to Stokes–Adams attacks and are treated with a pacemaker. ST segment elevation indicates ischaemia and irregularly irregular complexes are a feature of atrial fibrillation.

Woldemar Mobitz, Russian physician (1889-1951)

Karel Frederik Wenckebach, Dutch cardiologist (1864-1940)

43. Emergency management (2)

C. Intravenous lorazepam

In any situation it is essential that the patient's airway, breathing and circulation are intact before progressing to the management of any underlying condition. The first-line anti-epileptic medication used in seizures is intravenous lorazepam. It is important to have full resuscitation equipment available when administering intravenous benzodiazepines since there is a risk of respiratory arrest. If intravenous access is not possible, alternative options include rectal diazepam or buccal midazolam. If the benzodiazepines fail to stop the seizure, an intravenous infusion of phenytoin should be started. If this fails, an anaesthetist should be called to initiate general anaesthesia.

44. Supraventricular tachycardia

A. Administer adenosine

Supra-ventricular tachycardias are often paroxysmal and can last from seconds to hours. They can be caused by coffee, alcohol and tobacco but are usually the result of atrio-ventricular node (AVN) re-entry tachycardia (dual pathways within the AVN) or Wolff–Parkinson–White syndrome (an accessory atrio-ventricular pathway outside of the AVN). The narrow-complex tachycardia can exhaust a heart and precipitate failure due to inadequate filling during diastole, leading to reduced cardiac output. The Valsalva manoeuvre and carotid sinus massage can end this arrhythmia, as can cardioverting with adenosine (a very short-acting AV nodal blocking agent). For adenosine to work, it must be administered promptly: intravenous injection over 2 seconds via a large-bore cannula. The patient should continue to receive cardiac monitoring and the ward crash trolley should be close at hand as excessive atrio-ventricular node delay can lead to arrest.

Antonio Maria Valsalva, Italian physician (1666-1723)

45. Syndrome of inappropriate ADH secretion

D. Urine osmolality 800 mOsm/kg, plasma osmolality 250 mOsm/kg

This question should be simple to work out from first principles. If the syndrome features *inappropriate* ADH secretion (siADH), then the urine should be concentrated in the face of dilute plasma. By simple homeostatic principles, if the plasma is dilute, the urine should become more dilute in an attempt to concentrate the plasma. Option A, dilute urine with dilute plasma, could represent fluid overload. Option B, dilute urine with normal plasma concentration, could represent any cause of diuresis, which could become option C if the patient does not receive enough fluid intake! Option D shows concentrated urine but dilute plasma, consistent with siADH. Option E shows concentrated urine with concentrated plasma, which is most likely due to dehydration.

46. Systemic lupus erythematosus (3)

A. Acute pleuritis

Systemic lupus erythematosus is a chronic multisystem connective tissue disease of unknown cause. Almost 90% of affected individuals are women with a peak onset in the second and third decades. The patients present with myriad symptoms that could affect virtually every organ in the body. Constitutional symptoms such as fatigue, fever, and weight loss are present during the course of the disease, occurring in 50–100% of patients. Pleurisy, pleural effusion, pneumonitis, interstitial lung disease, pulmonary hypertension, and alveolar haemorrhage can all occur in SLE. In this case the presence of a friction rub and pleural effusion suggests the diagnosis of pleuritis. The pleural effusion in SLE is a mild exudate characterised by an elevation in pleural fluid low-dose heparin (LDH) but without signs of marked inflammation. Patients normally respond to therapy with non-steroidal anti-inflammatory drugs (NSAIDs), and moderate- to high-dose steroids are used if there is no response to NSAIDS within a few days.

47. Urinary frequency (2)

D. Hyperosmolar non-ketotic diabetic coma

Hyperosmolar non-ketotic diabetic coma (HONK) is a condition characterised by severe hyperglycaemia (>30–50 mmol/L) without significant hyperketonaemia or acidosis. It usually affects older patients, of which many have undiagnosed diabetes, or with past medical history of type 2 diabetes mellitus. In HONK the circulating insulin is sufficient to prevent ketogenesis but insufficient to allow the peripheral uptake and metabolism of glucose. As such the patient does not become acidotic. The hyperglycaemia causes an osmotic diuresis that rapidly dehydrates the patient and produces an extremely high plasma osmolality. There is hyperosmolality (>320 mOsm/kg) with severe dehydration, and pre-renal uraemia is common. The conscious level is depressed when plasma osmolarity is high, and the result is coma. These patients are usually sensitive to insulin and approximately 3 U/hour of insulin should be given initially. Excessive rates of fall of blood glucose (>5 mmol/hour) may be associated with cerebral oedema. Isotonic saline is given unless serum sodium exceeds 155 mmol/L, in which case 0.45% saline should be used. These patients have a high risk of deep vein thrombosis and thus prophylactic subcutaneous low molecular weight heparin is recommended. The mortality rate of HONK approaches 30%, which is likely to be a reflection of the advanced age of many of the patients and the presence of underlying illness.

48. Wilson's disease

B. Ask the patient to come in for an urgent blood test

Wilson's disease is an autosomal recessive disease of copper metabolism. In health, copper is transported in the serum bound to caeruloplasmin and is excreted in the bile. In Wilson's disease there is a defect in copper metabolism so it is not excreted in the bile and instead accumulates in the tissues. This process suppresses the synthesis of caeruloplasmin, which allows unbound (free) copper to enter the circulation. The high levels of free serum copper accumulate in vital organs such as the liver (cirrhosis), eye (Kayser–Fleischer rings), kidney and basal ganglia of the brain (personality changes). If left untreated the patient is at risk of developing cirrhosis, renal tubular disease, neurological disease and neuropsychiatric complications. Patients with Wilson's disease have an elevated serum free copper, urinary copper and hepatic copper (via biopsy). Paradoxically, total serum copper is usually low.

Penicillamine is used in the treatment of Wilson's disease as it chelates copper and other minerals and hence can prevent the deposition of copper into organs such as the liver and the central nervous system. Its use can reduce and help reverse pre-cirrhotic liver disease although neurological damage is often less reversible. It binds to circulating copper and facilitates its excretion in the urine. There are serious side effects of penicillamine, and patients should be advised to report any sore throat, temperatures or bruising. These signs may indicate agranulocytosis and immunosuppression that needs to be identified early, the drug stopped, and necessary action taken. Therefore, advising the patient to come in for an urgent blood test to look at the differential white cell count and the platelets would be the safest course of action. These severe reactions are dose-related but can occur early in the start of treatment, therefore regular blood testing is advisable following the commencement of penicillamine.

Samuel Alexander Wilson, British neurologist (1878-1937)

49. X-ray changes in osteoarthritis

C. Punched-out periarticular erosions

Osteoarthitis occurs when the articular cartilage has worn sufficiently to narrow the joint space and bring the bones together – increased friction and trauma between the bones causes the pain. Sclerosis and osteophytes are the bone's reaction to this increased friction and trauma which threatens to damage the bone. Subchondral cysts may also be seen on X-rays in osteoarthritis. "Punched out" periarticular erosions are more associated with gout.

50. Traveller's diarrhoea

B. *Escherichia coli*

E. coli infection can occur by spread through contaminated food and water supplies and it is the commonest cause of diarrhoea in the returning traveller. The other causes listed above should be suspected if diarrhoea is prolonged or there are other features such as mucus or blood in the stools. In prolonged causes of diarrhoea, parasitic infection such as *Giardia* should be tested for. Treatment is by rehydration, as *E. coli* gastroenteritis is a self-limiting condition. Patients should be educated about meticulous hand hygiene.

Index of Topics

Torsades de pointes, 66
Tremor, 151
Tuberculosis, 72, 73, 187, 223
Tumour markers, 122
Turner's syndrome, 219

Ulcerative colitis, 26, 191
Upper GI bleed, 61
Urinary tract infection, 223

Vertigo, 21
Vitamin B12 deficiency, 76
von Willebrand disease, 104

Warfarin therapy , 36, 180
Waterlow score, 105
Wegener's granulomatosis, 21
Wilson's disease, 240